JOINT COMMISSION

Framework *for* Improving Performance

From Principles to Practice

JOINT COMMISSION MISSION

The mission of the Joint Commission on Accreditation of Healthcare Organizations is to improve the quality of care provided to the public.

Printed in the U.S.A.

Requests for permission to reprint or make copies of any part of this work should be mailed to:
Permissions Editor
Department of Publications
Joint Commission on Accreditation of Healthcare Organizations

ISBN Number: 0-86688-364-9
Library of Congress Catalog Number: 94-75142

Contents

Introduction

This book, *Framework for Improving Performance: From Principles to Practice*, describes and exemplifies the Joint Commission's theory-based, practical methodology for continuously improving the core work and resulting outcomes of any health care organization. We believe that widespread adoption of this model will help organizations contribute to the central purpose of the health delivery system: to maximize the health of people served while conserving resources when that conservation does not jeopardize proper care of the patient.

WHAT IS THE ORIGIN OF THIS FRAMEWORK?

Driven by its mission "to improve the quality of health care provided to the public," the Joint Commission synthesized in this framework contemporary knowledge about a productive route to organizational excellence. This framework identifies the characteristics and behaviors of any health care organization striving to achieve high quality patient care, optimal patient outcomes, and efficient use of resources.

High quality care means that treatment of patients, residents, or clients is efficacious and appropriate. It is also available when needed, delivered in a timely fashion, and perceived by the patient to be provided in a manner that is respectful and caring. High quality care is also effective, safe, efficient, and coordinated over time and across practitioners and settings.

When a health care organization's performance exhibits these characteristics, positive results in the form of superior health outcomes, competitive costs, and high levels of satisfaction are much more likely. This is determined by how well critical systems, jobs, and tasks are carried out. Organizations that can provide empirical performance data about processes and outcomes are more likely to be seen favorably by patients and other relevant customers. This is the only sure route to future survival, success, and prosperity as a provider of choice. Also, a *performance-focused* accreditation process will greatly strengthen the partner-ship for quality between the Joint Commission and health care providers.

In developing this performance improvement framework, the Joint Commission has synthesized a wide range of theories, meth-ods, and tools. The framework has been shaped by systems think-ing, by performance measurement and assessment tools, by a functional rather than structural view of organizations, by process-mindedness, and by improvement knowledge. These resources give health care professionals the ability to systematically and scientifically enhance care processes and their outcomes.

In developing the framework, the Joint Commission has built upon the strengths of quality assurance and moved beyond its shortcomings. Quality assurance activities were too often frag-mented and compartmentalized, focused on retrospective inspec-tion and problem identification, and aimed at blaming individual clinicians. Remedies for these problems reside in strategies of total quality management (TQM) and continuous quality improvement (CQI). These strategies stress the importance of leadership, exter-nal and internal customers' needs, goal-driven design of new products and services, broad deployment of measurement systems, data-driven performance assessment, and systematic redesign of important organizational processes and functions.

WHAT ARE THE COMPONENTS OF THIS FRAMEWORK?

The framework for improving performance offers a broad perspective on organizational improvement. Although the Joint Commission is naturally most interested in its applicability to health care institutions, the theory and methods are relevant to any organization interested in continuous quality improvement. The framework addresses three issues which must be considered by any organization committed to excellence: its relationship to the external environment; its internal characteristics and functions; and a methodology for designing, measuring, assessing, and improving key functions or work processes.

The external environment. Critical success factors for health care organizations include the ability to understand and anticipate changes in the environment. Such changes include the demands of purchasers, payers, employers, regulators, consumers, and accrediting bodies for greater accountability. Health care reform efforts, laws, and standards are creating unpredictable changes. These changes and the increased competition are driving the creation of new organizational forms and the redesign of service delivery systems.

Successful organizations are flexible; they respond quickly to develop and implement new health services and delivery mechanisms. Such organizations are attuned to community needs and have an integrated approach to strategic planning, quality planning, and financial planning. Leaders of these organizations develop strategic plans that align the health care organization's mission with identified community needs.

The internal environment. Excellence in patient care clearly requires state-of-the-art professional knowledge, clinical expertise, and competence in technical skills. Furthermore, the knowledge, judgment, and skills among departments, disciplines, services, and units must be successfully coordinated and integrated to assure effective and efficient response to the needs of patients and their families.

The Joint Commission recognizes that the clinical functions that most influence patient outcomes, resource consumption, and patient satisfaction are rarely the responsibility of any single unit in an organization. This is evident in the transition from accreditation standards arranged by department, service, or structure to patient-focused standards dealing with the cross-disciplinary, multidepartmental functions most essential to patient care. The revised standards shift the focus from capability ("Is this institution organized logically to do its jobs?") to performance ("Are the key processes in this institution carried out well so that optimal results are achieved?").

Clinical management of patients is a central component of a health care organization's performance objectives. However, governance, management of the organization, and support activities are equally important to the organizational *system*. Four pivotal functions in the internal environment of a health care organization are the performance of leaders, the management of human resources, the management of information, and the continuous improvement of performance and outcomes.

Leaders must define a strategic plan that is consistent with the organization's mission and vision. They must communicate this plan throughout the organization and allocate sufficient resources to accomplish the primary goals. Other responsibilities of health care leaders include building teamwork, fostering constant learning, encouraging risk taking, as well as coaching and enabling staff to acquire the knowledge and skills needed to improve processes and outputs.

Effective management of human resources helps ensure that adequate numbers of staff and licensed independent practitioners are available when and where needed, that they are competent to carry out their processes and meet the needs of those who depend on them, and that their performance is assessed and improved through continuing education. Recognition and reward mechanisms must be examined to be sure they are promoting collaborative, patient-minded behaviors.

A well-designed, well-functioning information management system provides timely, reliable, and accurate information to support data-based decision making. Such a system enables staff to coordinate, integrate, measure, and improve their work.

Finally, continuous improvement and constant striving for higher quality must be an integral component of the organization's mission, vision of the future, value system, and daily work. Input and feedback from patients, staff, and other key customers should guide the improvement process. Breaking down barriers (including turf boundaries) to enhance communication is an essential prerequisite for teamwork in service delivery, problem solving, and innovation. Successful organizations focus improvement efforts on fixing systems, not on searching out and punishing alleged dysfunctional individuals.

WHAT IS THE CYCLE FOR IMPROVING PERFORMANCE?

The third element of the framework for improving performance is a methodology that describes in practical, operational terms how to systematically and scientifically improve the important functions of a health care organization. The performance improvement cycle is not a recent invention; improving performance and patient outcomes have always been at the core of Joint Commission accreditation.

The cycle outlines essential activities common to a variety of improvement approaches and allows organizations a great deal of flexibility in how they implement their design, measurement, assessment, and improvement work. It is a logical enhancement to former quality assurance methods and is better anchored in the real work of health care professionals and in real benefits for patients and others.

The performance improvement cycle is an ongoing process. An organization may reasonably initiate its improvement effort at any point in the cycle by

- defining objectives for a new service and designing the delivery system;
- flowcharting existing clinical or administrative processes and measuring their results;
- comparing its performance to that of other institutions;
- analyzing data and selecting areas for priority attention; or
- brainstorming and experimenting with new patient care or support processes.

The cycle is not composed of sequential steps; often several components will be underway simultaneously.

The "Improving Organizational Performance" standards in the 1994 *Accreditation Manual for Hospitals* (and scheduled for all other manuals in 1995 and 1996) define the activities necessary to improve everyday functions and processes. The improvement cycle is applicable at many levels: to the organization as a whole; at the level of cross-departmental, multidisciplinary functions (such as patient education or medication use); at the level of specific processes (such as pain assessment, renal dialysis, or personnel recruitment); or at the level of concrete tasks (such as drawing arterial blood, labeling and transporting specimens, or scheduling clinic appointments).

Design refers to the deliberate process of creating a quality service from the recipient's perspective. Designing or planning is a goal-driven activity that seeks ways to build quality characteristics such as efficacy, appropriateness, timeliness, safety, and respect into the process.

Health care processes or functions are typically carried out by interdependent teams whose work and results are the subject of routine, ongoing measurement as well as time-limited, focused data collection. A well-balanced measurement system addresses multiple dimensions of performance, collects data about processes, outcomes, resource consumption, and satisfaction levels, and taps into patient, practitioner, and employee views on quality. Performance data assembled in an internal database or compared to an external reference database must be evaluated or critically analyzed by "process owners" and leaders. Quality improvement tools are often helpful for interpreting variation in processes or outcomes and for conducting an analysis to discover the root cause of a problem. The purpose of this assessment is to draw conclusions about current performance and then decide whether to pursue an opportunity for improvement or resolution of a problem.

Privilege delineation, peer review processes, or performance appraisal mechanisms may be involved when the competence of individual practitioners, staff members, or employees is in question.

Once priority topics having potential significant benefits to patient care are identified, a systematic, empirical improvement/innovation activity is launched. Whether it is called the scientific method or the Shewhart/Deming/PDCA/PDSA cycle, this work involves planning an improvement, implementing the new approach (usually on a pilot basis), collecting and analyzing data about its impact, and taking action to standardize a successful process innovation. The PDSA cycle can be repeated if results are not satisfactory.

The outcome of an improvement project is the redesign of an existing function or process. If the PDSA cycle focuses on innovation, then the design of a new function or process results. In either case, the cycle for improving performance provides a more effective way to meet patients' needs, or even to exceed their expectations.

SUMMARY

This performance improvement framework incorporates several key assertions:

- Performance means *what* is done and *how well it is done*—for example, what jobs are done to provide health care and how effectively they are carried out. Joint Commission standards manuals are being reorganized to address the most important governance, management, clinical, and support functions.
- The organization's performance of these functions is reflected in patient outcomes, in the cost (or efficiency) of its services, and in patients' and others' satisfaction.
- Patients and others judge the quality of health care based on health outcomes (and sometimes on their experiences of the care process and level of service provided).
- Patients, purchasers, regulators, and other stakeholders expect and use quantitative/explicit data and qualitative/implicit perceptions to judge quality and value of health care.

The framework for improving performance describes a global model for organizations in pursuit of excellence. Its three components—external environment, internal environment, and operational improvement methodology—are not a cookbook of required activities. Rather, they are a synthesis of important concepts, organizational characteristics, management skills, and scientific tools and techniques that together make continuous improvement possible.

This improvement framework should lead to many challenges for health care organizations. These challenges include becoming more patient-focused, redesigning care processes, promoting collaborative teamwork, systematically measuring and assessing performance, and encouraging risk taking and experimentation. Nonetheless, the ability to proactively and effectively manage quality is the only way that organizations will survive and prosper in the face of stringent resource constraints and increasing demands for better health outcomes.

The Joint Commission is firm in its conviction that this framework for improving performance enhances all of our abilities as committed, conscientious health care professionals to do better on behalf of our patients.

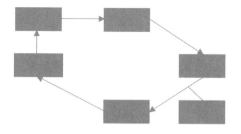

Chapter 1
OVERVIEW

Today, we need go no further than the local newspaper or a television news broadcast to see the intense concern about the future of health care: its availability, its quality, and most particularly, its cost. These pervasive concerns—shared by patients, health care providers, the public, purchasers, payers, accreditors, regulators, and others—are fueling unprecedented efforts to understand and improve how health care is delivered.

For over 40 years, the Joint Commission has pursued a mission that is perhaps more critical today than ever. That mission is *to improve the quality of care provided to the public.* The Joint Commission has carried out this mission through several ongoing activities:

- Gaining national consensus on standards for health care organizations;
- Evaluating organizations to determine compliance with the standards;

- Educating health care organizations about performance improvement and other issues central to quality; and
- Developing indicators useful to organizations and the Joint Commission in evaluating the level of performance of important health care functions.

The missions of the Joint Commission and the health care organizations seeking its accreditation are aligned. The Joint Commission and health care organizations are driven to improve the quality of care provided to the public.

This book describes one product of the Joint Commission's activities in pursuit of its mission: a *framework for improving performance*. The framework is a flexible, practical approach to improving performance; it synthesizes a range of important concepts and methods and can be used by a variety of health care organizations, including hospitals, health care networks, mental health facilities, long term care facilities, home care organizations, and ambulatory care organizations. The framework has these primary goals:

- To emphasize that an organization's performance of important functions significantly affects its patient outcomes, the costs to achieve these outcomes, and judgments about the quality and value of its services;
- To illustrate how an organization can mesh the rich variety of concepts and methods developed independently over the last several decades into an operational performance improvement system; and
- To show how the effectiveness with which an organization manages its relationships with the external environment is equally important to the fulfillment of its mission as the effectiveness with which it manages its internal environment.

This book explains this framework for improving performance and shows how it can be put into operation. Initially, we provide an overview of the principles and history on which the framework is built, and introduce the primary components of the framework which include

- the external environment, including the political, social, economic, and other forces in society that a health care organization must address to fulfill its mission;

- the internal environment, particularly those important governance, management, clinical, and support activities that affect patient care and outcomes; and
- the cycle for improving performance—a practical method for improving processes.

Subsequent chapters explore each stage of the improvement cycle, answering the core questions about each activity and presenting examples adapted from experiences of health care organizations around the country.

This book is intended as a practical guide. It can be used to acquire an overview of performance improvement concepts and methods, and it can be used as a reference tool to help organizations carry out their improvement activities. The book also contains three helpful appendixes: 1) the Joint Commission's "Improving Organizational Performance" standards, 2) excerpts from the scoring guidelines that explain and interpret these standards, and 3) indicators being developed for the Joint Commission's indicator measurement system. (The "Improving Organization Performance" standards follow the basic parts of the cycle for improving performance: design, measure, assess, and improve.)

With that preface, we can proceed to build the foundation that underlies the framework for improving performance.

I. UNDERLYING PRINCIPLES

This framework for improving performance rests on several related principles about the purpose of health care, how health care is provided, and how health care is improved. To clarify our foundation, we will briefly state the principles here. In the remaining chapters, the principles can be seen in practice.

The Purpose of Health Care

The focus of health care is the people it serves, regardless of the specific setting or service. Whether in-hospital acute care, ambulatory care, home care, mental health care, or long term care, the central purpose of health care is to maximize the health of the people served while conserving resources, when that conservation does not jeopardize proper care of the patient.

The purpose of health care—especially in today's environment—encompasses not only patient health outcomes, but also efficient resource use to achieve those outcomes. The value of care depends on the balance of outcomes achieved and resources used.

This framework is designed to help health care organizations pursue the goal of cost-effective care—optimal patient outcomes at the lowest possible cost.

Dimensions of Performance

Patient outcomes and resource use are strongly affected by nine important dimensions of the performance of a health care organization. To patients and others, these are also dimensions of the quality of health care they receive. The advantage of focusing on these dimensions of performance is that they can be measured and improved—progress can be tracked. The nine dimensions encompass the following:

- the *efficacy* of a procedure or treatment for a specific condition;
- the *appropriateness* of a specific test, procedure, or service to meet a patient's needs;
- the *availability* of a needed test, procedure, treatment, or service to a patient who needs it;
- the *effectiveness* with which tests, procedures, treatments, and services are provided;
- the *timeliness* with which a needed test, procedure, treatment, or service is provided to a patient;
- the *safety* to the patient, staff, and others involved in the services provided;
- the *efficiency* with which services are provided;
- the *continuity* of the services provided to a patient with respect to other services, other practitioners, and other providers, and over time.
- the *respect and caring* with which services are provided.

These dimensions of performance are further defined in Table 1-1 on page 17.

Table 1-1. Dimensions of Performance

I. Doing the Right Thing

The *efficacy* of the procedure or treatment in relation to the patient's condition.
> The degree to which the care/intervention for the patient has been shown to accomplish the desired/projected outcome(s).

The *appropriateness* of a specific test, procedure, or service to meet the patient's needs.
> The degree to which the care/intervention provided is relevant to the patient's clinical needs, given the current state of the art.

II. Doing the Right Thing Well

The *availability* of a needed test, procedure, treatment, or service to the patient who needs it.
> The degree to which appropriate care/intervention is available to meet the patient's needs.

The *effectiveness* with which tests, procedures, treatments, and services are provided.
> The degree to which the care/intervention is provided in the correct manner, given the current state of the art, in order to achieve the desired/projected outcome for the patient.

The *timeliness* with which a needed test, procedure, treatment, or service is provided to the patient.
> The degree to which the care/intervention is provided to the patient at the most beneficial or necessary time.

The *safety* to the patient, staff, and customers (and others) involved in the services provided.
> The degree to which the risk of an intervention and risk in the care environment are reduced for the patient and health care provider.

The *efficiency* with which services are provided.
> The ratio of the outcomes (results of care) for a patient to the resources used to deliver the care.

The *continuity* of the services provided to the patient with respect to other services, practitioners, and other providers, and over time.
> The degree to which the care/intervention for the patient is coordinated among practitioners, among organizations, and across time.

The *respect and caring* with which services are provided.
> The degree to which the patient, or designee, is involved in his or her own care decisions, and to which those persons providing services do so with sensitivity and respect for the patient's needs, expectations, and individual differences.

Functions and Processes

The degree to which health care fulfills the nine dimensions of performance is strongly influenced by the design and operation of a series of important functions (see Table 1-2, page 19). In health care, examples of functions include direct patient care activities (such as patient assessment, treatment, and patient/family education), as well as governance, management, and support services (such as management of information and management of human resources).

A *function* is a group of processes with a common goal. A *process* is a series of linked, goal-directed activities. For example, we might view information management as a function and data entry as a process within that function, or we might view medication use as a function and medication administration as a process within that function.

The framework for improving performance views the processes involved in providing care and services to patients in health care organizations not as isolated tasks, but as a series of activities linked to form important functions. The framework focuses on the design, measurement, assessment, and improvement of these functions as well as of the processes within them. The framework is not limited to direct patient care functions, but recognizes that governance, management, and support functions are also key influences on health outcomes.

All Joint Commission's standards manuals are undergoing reorganization to reflect these important functions. Table 1-3, page 20, shows the organization of the 1994 *Accreditation Manual for Hospitals.* The standards are divided into three sections: care of the patient (functions primarily involving direct and indirect patient care), organizational functions (functions carried out throughout the organization that do not primarily involve direct patient care), and structures with important functions (governing body, management, medical staff, and nursing). Upcoming manuals for mental health care, ambulatory care, long term care, home care, and health care networks will also be based on important patient care and organizational functions.

This process- and function-focused view of an organization has several important implications for improving organizational perfor-

Table 1-2. Health Care Functions

Those systems, processes, or jobs that most directly and tangibly affect patient outcomes.

1. **Caring for the patient**
   - Clinical activities

2. **Managing the organization**
   - Governance
   - Administration
   - Support services

mance. These implications underlie most of the activities described in this book.

- **Crossing organizational boundaries.** Most work in health care organizations is accomplished by teams of interdependent staff. Their individual efforts must be coordinated to achieve common goals. These goals cannot be accomplished unless processes and communication can freely cross intra-organizational boundaries. Different disciplines and different levels of staff must be able to communicate effectively. In a specific design or improvement effort, for example, one discipline alone will not be able to implement a process that involves several disciplines.

- **Customer-supplier relationships.** Work is completed by enacting a series of customer-supplier relationships or "hand-offs." Well-designed processes better facilitate these hand-offs. An organization has internal customers and suppliers (for example, physicians and pharmacists in the prescription process) and external customers (for example, major employers) and suppliers (for example, pharmaceutical companies, equipment vendors).

- **Outcomes.** Every process, by definition, produces results. These results may be intended and desirable, unintended and desirable, or unintended and undesirable. To determine how a process is performing, an organization must measure not only the activities involved in the process, but also the outcomes it produces.

Table 1-3 Important Functions Identified in the 1994 Accreditation Manual for Hospitals

Care of the Patient
- Rights of patients and organizational ethics
- Assessment of patients
- Treatment of patients
  - Medication use
  - Operative and other invasive procedures
  - Nutritional care
- Education of patients and family
- Coordination of care, including entry to setting or service

Organizational Functions
- Leadership
- Management of information
- Management of human resources
- Management of the environment of care
- Surveillance, prevention, and control of infection
- Improving organizational performance

Structures with Important Functions
- Governing body
- Management and administration
- Medical staff
- Nursing

- *Variation in processes and outcomes.* Variation in all processes—and, therefore, in their outcomes—is normal. Observing and measuring this variation triggers a search for explanations. Analyzing the causes of variation helps distinguish between a special cause (nonrecurring event) and a common or systemic cause, and is an effective means of improving the performance of functions and processes.

- *Processes rather than individuals.* Ordinarily, designing or improving a process to achieve performance goals is best accomplished by focusing on the process rather than on the individuals who carry out the process. Occasionally a lack of knowledge, skill, judgment, or motivation of an individual will result in undesirable performance. Most opportunities for improvement, however, reside in processes.

Outcomes, Cost, Quality, and Value

The effect of an organization's performance of important functions can be viewed in various ways:

- In its patient outcomes;
- In the cost of its services;
- In the satisfaction of patients and others with the outcomes and the way they were achieved; and
- In the judgments important customers, including patients, make about the quality and value of care provided.

(Figure 1-1, page 22, illustrates the relationship between performance, results, and judgments about quality and value.) The framework described in this book focuses on improving the results of health care (including the outcomes of care) and on improving judgments about the quality and value of the health care.

Improving Performance

Outcomes, satisfaction, quality, and value can be enhanced by systematically designing, measuring, assessing, and improving the organization's functions (such as medication use, operative and other invasive procedures, management of information), and the processes within the functions (such as emergency drug delivery, total hip replacement, billing). This framework, including its core component—the cycle for improving performance—combines various methods to carry out these systematic activities. These methods share the belief that opportunities for overall improvement most often lie in the design and implementation of organizational functions and processes, rather than in the scrutiny of an individual's performance.

II. A BRIEF HISTORY OF QUALITY ASSESSMENT AND IMPROVEMENT IN HEALTH CARE

Health care has a diverse history of quality initiatives, ranging from early efforts to measure outcomes to medical audits to practice guidelines to total quality management. The framework for improving performance draws on the most successful approaches to improvement; it synthesizes those approaches into a logical and flexible cycle to carry out a wide range of improvement activities.

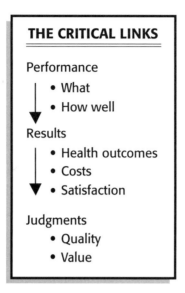

Figure 1-1. *This illustration shows the important links between performance, outcomes, and judgments of quality and value. This concept is one rationale for focusing this framework on performance.*

This section reviews some of health care's most notable improvement efforts and provides a context for the framework described in this book. Figure 1-2, page 24, illustrates this evolution of approaches.

Quality Assurance

In the early part of this century, Dr Ernest Codman advocated routine collection and publication of patient outcome data; he believed these data should be used to assess and improve the quality of patient care. Although his specific proposals were not accepted, they did influence the initial hospital accreditation standards. The "Minimum Standard" of the American College of Surgeons' Hospital Standardization Program stated that the medical staff should "review and analyze at regular intervals their clinical experience in the various departments of the hospital."[1]

The activities now known as quality assurance are derived from this requirement in the Minimum Standard. The requirement has evolved from its initial form (implicit peer-based discussions) through retrospective time-limited audits (in the 1970s) to its current form: ongoing monitoring, evaluation, and improvement using well-chosen process and outcome indicators.

Embedded in this evolution is the enduring, but mistaken, belief that patient outcomes are affected solely by the patient's severity of illness and the quality of direct hands-on care. This belief implies that the nature and quality of governance and management activities have minimal effect on patient outcomes.

This conceptual framework has led to placing quality assurance activities within the clinical structures of health care organizations (for example, medical staff services, nursing services, pharmaceutical services, and so on). Within this context, growing professional specialization has had an unintended side-effect: quality assurance activities have become increasingly fragmented. This has happened because quality assurance activities have been carried out as isolated activities in separate services and disciplines. Such uncoordinated measurement, assessment, and improvement activities have ignored the fact that health care organizations are and must be treated as coordinated systems.

In the 1980s, the effectiveness of improvement efforts was further undermined by a growing tendency to blame identified problems on individual practitioners or providers, alleging deficiencies in knowledge, skill, or judgment. Thus, quality assurance became a punitive, problem-focused policing mechanism unwelcome by the clinicians on whom it focused. The fragmented nature of quality assurance, coupled with its increasingly punitive connotations, prompted a search for more productive approaches to measuring, assessing, and improving health care.

Research Activities

While quality assurance was evolving within hospital services and other provider organizations, new measurement and assessment tools were emerging from health services research. This work began quietly in the 1960s and 1970s, and it exploded in the 1980s. In large part, the explosion was a response to the growing awareness of significant variations in practices and patient outcomes. The work was facilitated by the rapid evolution of informa-

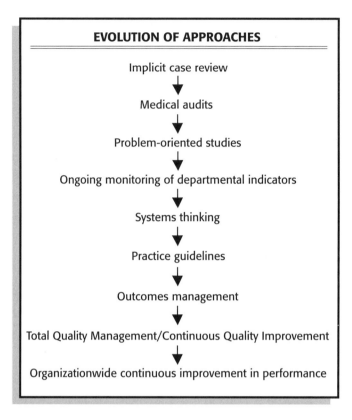

Figure 1-2. *Approaches to health care assessment and improvement have evolved considerably since early this century, with the most intensive activity coming in the past ten years.*

tion technology, which made the creation and use of large databases possible.

The tools resulting from this work include the following:

- an expanded library of process and outcome indicators, as well as functional status and patient satisfaction measures;
- clinical practice guidelines/parameters, clinical algorithms, and critical paths;
- the tracking of patient health outcomes by an organization for its own improvement and the aggregation of patient health outcomes from many organizations to develop evidence-based practice guidelines; and

- reference databases containing process and outcome data from multiple health care organizations.

(Development of process and outcome indicators is exemplified by the Joint Commission's activities in this area, discussed in Chapter 3.)

During the late 1980s, a small but growing number of quality assurance programs began to use these tools.

Total Quality Management/Continuous Quality Improvement

A third approach to improving health care is derived from the theories and methodologies of total quality management (TQM) and continuous quality improvement (CQI). Although this approach exists in many varieties, the following characteristics are common to most versions:

- ***Central role of leaders.*** Leaders understand and emphasize the strategic importance of high-quality products and services.
- ***Environment of respect and empowerment.*** Organizations create an environment that enables each individual to contribute to the organization's objectives and to enhance his or her knowledge and skills.
- ***Customer expectations.*** The customer is the preeminent definer and judge of the quality and value of the organization's products and services.
- ***Systematic design.*** New products and services are designed in a planned, systematic fashion to assure that procedures are effective and efficient, and that the resulting service or product meets the known requirements of the customers.
- ***Measurement systems.*** Systems to measure processes and outcomes are carefully developed and widely deployed.
- ***Data collection and analysis.*** Improvement efforts are based on data that have been carefully collected and analyzed using various statistical tools.
- ***Systematic redesign.*** Products and services are systematically redesigned to improve their quality and value and to reduce the time and resources needed for development and production.

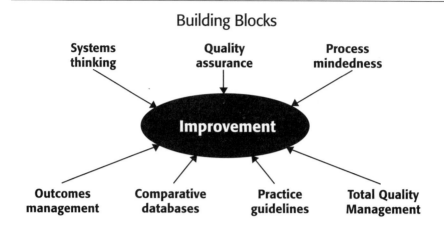

Figure 1-3. *This figure shows how the Joint Commission's framework for improving performance synthesizes parts of many approaches to design, measurement, assessment, and improvement.*

Systems theory did not originate with TQM/CQI. Modern-day systems thinking evolved from the general systems theory foundation of the 1950s. This theory helped us understand that an organization is a system whose individual parts must work well together if performance, patient outcomes, quality, and value are to be maximized. By highlighting the interdependent nature of a health care organization's work, those involved in systems theory have encouraged cross-functional teamwork at all levels. This teamwork is essential to effectively apply the process design, measurement, assessment, and improvement tools now available.

Figure 1-3 illustrates some of the more important concepts and methods that have been incorporated into the framework for improving performance.

III. FRAMEWORK FOR IMPROVING PERFORMANCE

The framework for improving performance offers a broad perspective on improvement. It recognizes the range of external issues (such as health care reform and community needs) that affect an organization's performance. It also recognizes the range of issues inside an organization (such as leadership and human resources) that affect performance. Finally, it presents an adaptable cycle for

Framework for Improving Performance

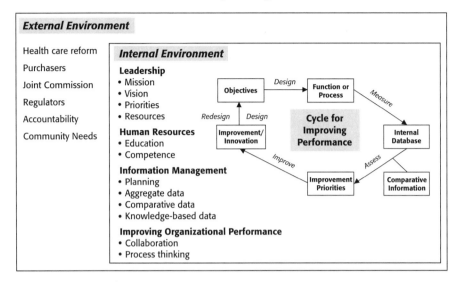

Figure 1-4. *This illustration depicts the three core components of the framework for improving performance: external environment, internal environment, and cycle for improving performance.*

designing, measuring, assessing, and improving processes and outcomes in a health care organization. This framework reflects what the Joint Commission believes an organization committed to excellence must minimally address.

Figure 1-4 illustrates this framework's three basic components:

- External environment;
- Internal environment; and
- Cycle for improving performance.

The following sections introduce each of these components.

External Environment

By external environment, we mean the factors outside a health care organization that affect the way the organization designs and carries out its services (see Figure 1-5, page 28). Organizations striving to excel are continuously surveying their environment, eliciting feedback from customers and others, and acting accordingly. Today, health care organizations must monitor and address

Framework for Improving Performance—
External Environment

External Environment

Health care reform

Purchasers

Joint Commission

Regulators

Accountability

Community Needs

Figure 1-5. *This figure illustrates issues present in the external environment that drive the design and delivery of health care.*

at least the following forces for change:

- *Health care reform*—the need to prepare for a possible recon-figuration in the health care delivery and payment system.
- *Purchasers*—the need to address purchaser's expectations of value and quality.
- *The Joint Commission*—the need to meet nationally recognized standards.
- *Regulators*—the need to fulfill regulatory requirements, which affect the design of many services.
- *Accountability*—the need to demonstrate to others (including patients, the community, and purchasers) the quality and value of the health care provided.
- *Community needs*—the need to understand and address the needs and expectations of the community served.

The framework for improving performance urges organizations to recognize how such factors in the external environment interact with the organization's internal environment and performance improvement efforts.

Framework for Improving Performance—
Internal Environment

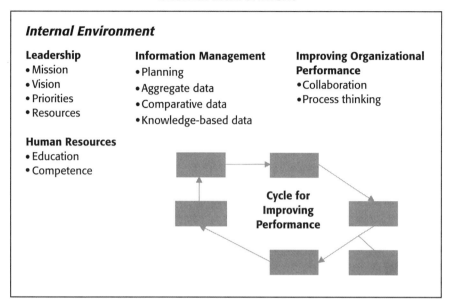

Internal Environment

Leadership
• Mission
• Vision
• Priorities
• Resources

Information Management
• Planning
• Aggregate data
• Comparative data
• Knowledge-based data

Improving Organizational Performance
• Collaboration
• Process thinking

Human Resources
• Education
• Competence

Cycle for
Improving
Performance

Figure 1-6. *This figure shows factors in the internal health care environment that affect performance.*

Internal Environment

"Internal environment" is a blanket term for the functions inside an organization that most influence performance. This includes its design, measurement, assessment, and improvement of processes (see Figure 1-6). The following internal functions are most important in determining the overall quality and value of the care and other services provided by a health care organization:

• leadership;

• management of human resources;

• management of information; and

• improvement of organizational performance.

Leadership. Leaders must define a strategic plan that is consistent with the organization's mission and vision, communicate this plan (and the mission and vision) throughout the organization, and allocate resources to accomplish the plan's goals.

Other leadership activities can have enormous influence on

organizational performance. Building teamwork and fostering continuous improvement often require leaders to become better facilitators and coaches, to foster constant learning, and to encourage innovation and risk taking. Leaders also encourage continuous improvement through their personal involvement in measurement, assessment, and improvement activities—especially as they apply to the leadership process itself.

"Empowerment" is another concept gaining currency among leaders. Many effective leaders enable or empower staff throughout the organization to acquire and apply the knowledge and skills to continuously improve processes and services.

Leaders in a health care organization include at least the leaders of the governing body; the chief executive officer and other senior managers; the elected and/or appointed leaders of the medical staff and the clinical departments and other medical staff members in hospital administrative positions; and the nurse executive and other senior nursing leaders. Effective leaders share certain qualities:

- Expertise in their areas of responsibility;
- Knowledge about improvement, including an understanding of systems, variation, measurement, and the psychology of human behavior and motivation;
- Authority and willingness to allocate resources in the service of continuous improvement;
- An understanding that improvement is essential to an organization's success and survival; and
- A passion for improvement.

Leaders are the driving force behind the other functions of the internal environment, in addition to being a major influence in the way an organization responds to the external environment.

Management of human resources. For an organization to fulfill its objectives (including the objective of continuous improvement) it must have adequate numbers of competent staff available to carry out all key governance, management, clinical, and support processes. Their performance must be regularly assessed and improved through continuing education and training opportunities.

Management of information. Health care depends on timely, valid, and reliable information about

- the science of health care delivery;
- individual patients, their care, and its results;
- administrative and business functions;
- performance of the organization as a whole; and
- from external reference databases, other organizations' performance.

Meeting these information needs is essential if an organization is going to coordinate, integrate, assess, and improve its services.

Improving organizational performance. Another characteristic of organizations striving to excel is that they are rigorous and diligent in analyzing their results and in using that self-evaluation to generate improvement. This function includes activities that create well-designed processes, measure the performance of existing processes, assess processes based on measurement data, and improve outcomes by redesigning existing processes or by designing new processes when necessary. The Joint Commission's current "Improving Organizational Performance" standards—like the framework described in this book—accommodates a variety of process improvement methodologies. Certain key concepts are common to almost all performance improvement approaches:

- It is essential to consider patients' and others' judgments about quality and their view of the need for improvement.
- Close coordination and collaboration are necessary among departments, services, and disciplines.
- Improvement opportunities usually lie in processes, not in an individual's performance deficiencies.

It is worthwhile to briefly expand on this last concept. The vast majority of individuals are intrinsically motivated to perform well and help their organization achieve its goals. This philosophy contrasts sharply with the punitive connotation of quality assurance. The respect that emerges from this tenet could revive practitioner involvement in patient-oriented measurement, assessment, and improvement efforts.

Cycle for Improving Performance

As part of its internal environment, an organization must have a core process for systematic improvement. This process improvement methodology merges the design, measurement, assessment, and improvement tools, allowing those tools to be put to effective, continuous use. The cycle for improving performance—the third component of this framework—describes a systematic approach to such a process. Figure 1-7, page 33, illustrates this cycle. The explanation that follows refers to this illustration.

The cyclical nature of this approach to improvement suggests

- it is continuous; and
- improvement work can, and actually does, begin at any point in the cycle.

To improve processes and outcomes over time, staff of health care organizations must systematically and scientifically

- design;
- measure;
- assess;
- improve; and
- design/redesign.

The boxes in Figure 1-7 describe the building blocks of the improvement cycle:

- *Objectives* for achieving a clear goal or purpose are necessary before launching a design effort.
- A design effort results in a *function or process*—a related series of activities directed toward accomplishing a specific goal.
- Measuring performance of a function or process results in an *internal database*, which is used to assess performance over time.
- One of the tools used to assess performance is *comparative information* from other sources, such as reference databases and practice guidelines.
- Assessment of a process should result in identifying *opportunities for improvement* and setting *priorities* among them.
- Based on these priorities, the organization creates, tests, and implements specific *improvements and innovations*, which involve redesign or a new design, respectively, of a process or function.

Cycle for Improving Performance

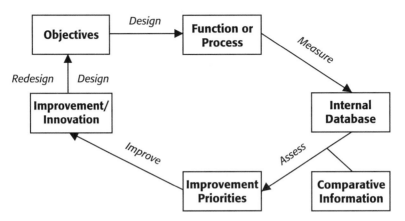

Figure 1-7. *This cycle is composed of activities (the lines and words above them) and the inputs to and outputs from the activities (in boxes). The cycle is continuous and can be entered at any point.*

It is important to note that once an organization has completed this cycle for a given function or process, the cycle continues. The objectives are reviewed and perhaps changed. Measurement continues in order to determine whether improvement has occurred and is sustained. The internal database continues to grow. And assessment using the ever-growing information base may identify further opportunities for improvement.

This cycle is anchored in the real work of an organization—the functions and processes it carries out every day to pursue goals, narrow and broad.

This cycle can be carried out by existing workgroups as part of everyday activities. When the process or function being addressed crosses unit or departmental boundaries, however, it may be necessary to identify or form a specific team composed of the people who are responsible for the process, who carry out the process, and who are affected by the process.

The improvement cycle may be applied at any level of generality or specificity. For example, "function" can refer to the entire health care organization as a complex system, or "function" can refer to a multidisciplinary, cross-service activity such as patient

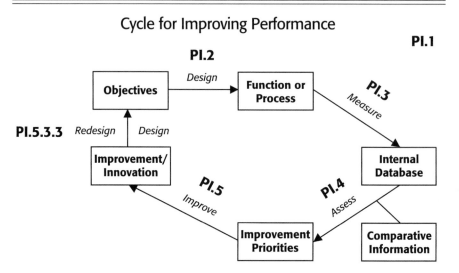

Figure 1-8. *This version of the improvement cycle shows the relationship of each step to the "Improving Organizational Performance" standards in the 1994* Accreditation Manual for Hospitals.

assessment. "Process" can refer to the specific steps for labeling specimens for transport from an extended care facility or home to the laboratory. "Process" can also refer to how pneumonia patients are treated or how total hip replacement is carried out. Finally, "process" can refer to how ambulatory patients are scheduled for clinic appointments or the organized way intakes for individuals with mental health problems are completed.

Subsequent chapters of this book will provide a more in-depth explanation of how to carry out this cycle.

Relationship of the Cycle to the Joint Commission's Standards

The cycle for improving organizational performance is the basis of the Joint Commission's "Improving Organizational Performance" standards. These standards and excerpts from the scoring guidelines are reprinted in Appendixes A and B of this book. The standards, like the cycle, focus primarily on the performance of an organization's systems and processes, not solely on performance of individuals. Figure 1-8 shows which "Improving Organizational Performance" standards apply to which parts of the cycle.

IV. SUMMARY POINTS

- *Underlying principles.*
  - The purpose of health care is to maximize patient health and to use resources efficiently and appropriately.
  - Patient outcomes and resource use are strongly affected by the following nine measurable dimensions of performance: efficacy, appropriateness, availability, effectiveness, timeliness, safety, efficiency, continuity, and respect and caring.
  - The degree to which health care fulfills these nine dimensions of performance is strongly influenced by the design and operation of a series of important functions.
  - The effect of an organization's performance of its important functions is evident in patient outcomes, in satisfaction with its services, in the cost of its services, and in the judgments about the quality and value of these services made by the organization and others.
- *The approaches to and tools of health care improvement have evolved.* These now include
  - quality assurance;
  - practice guidelines;
  - process mindedness;
  - outcomes management/comparative databases;
  - total quality management/continuous quality improvement; and
  - systems thinking.
- *The framework for improving performance* incorporates various concepts and methods into a flexible approach to improvement. The framework has three basic components:
  - External environment, including the political, social, economic, and other forces in society that a health care organization must address to fulfill its mission;
  - Internal environment, particularly those important governance, management, clinical, and support activities that effect patient care and outcomes; and
  - Cycle for improving performance, a practical method for improving processes.

REFERENCES

1. Roberts JS, Coale J, Redman RR: A history of the Joint Commission. *JAMA* 7: 936-940, August, 1987.

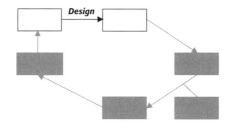

Chapter 2
DESIGN

Transporting a patient from the operating room to the intensive care unit...phoning a home care client to schedule a visit...creating a treatment plan for a chemical dependency patient...prescribing a medication...implementing a computerized information system...establishing an infrastructure for performance improvement....No activity, process, or function in a health care organization is an end in itself. All should be logical parts of a larger whole. In other words, they should be designed to fulfill an objective.

At the organizational level, at the department, unit, or team level, and at the individual level, we need to regularly stop and ask ourselves two questions:

- What goals are we trying to accomplish?
- How can we best accomplish those goals?

Cycle for Improving Performance—Design

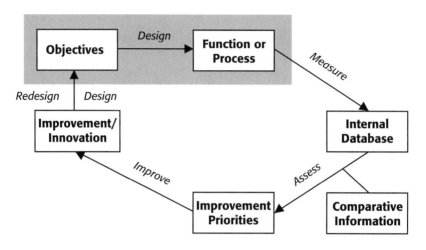

Figure 2-1. *This figure highlights the* **design** *stage of the improvement cycle—the subject of this chapter.*

These questions encapsulate the concept of design. Figure 2-1 shows how design fits into the cycle for improving performance. In this cycle, design means

- determining the objectives toward which an organization's activities aim; and
- designing and implementing functions and processes to achieve those objectives.

Figure 2-2, page 39, shows some of the issues involved in determining objectives and designing and implementing functions and processes.

Before proceeding further, it is important to distinguish between *design* and *redesign*. Design means creating new processes—in effect, starting with a clean slate. Redesign means taking a fresh look at an existing process—in effect, revising and improving the process. Although many of the same techniques apply to both (for example, reviewing state-of-the-art knowledge about the process), some important distinctions exist as well. For example, in redesign, an organization would most likely use information about its current performance of the process as part of the effort. An organization creating a new design would not

Cycle for Improving Performance—Design Issues

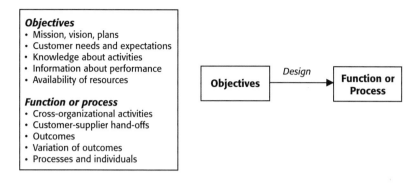

Objectives
- Mission, vision, plans
- Customer needs and expectations
- Knowledge about activities
- Information about performance
- Availability of resources

Function or process
- Cross-organizational activities
- Customer-supplier hand-offs
- Outcomes
- Variation of outcomes
- Processes and individuals

Figure 2-2. *These issues influence the two components of process design: setting objectives and designating functions and processes.*

have that information to use, because the process would not yet exist.

This chapter focuses primarily on new design. It is intended for organizations that may be, for example, building a new facility, extending a product line (such as, moving from diagnostic arteriography to cardiovascular angioplasty), or offering a new clinical service (such as a chronic pain clinic).

I. WHY DO WE DESIGN? SETTING OBJECTIVES

Successful health care delivery is driven by goals, both narrow and broad. For example, an activity such as scheduling a follow-up appointment for positive test results has a range of goals from reaching the individual on the telephone to facilitating an examination to serving the patient's health needs. Unfortunately, many goals are often unexpressed (unwritten and unspoken). All goals should regularly be examined to determine whether

- they continue to be relevant and valuable;
- they can be met by the activities and processes in place;
- they are being effectively and efficiently pursued; and
- any new ones should be established.

Development of an organization's goals (from the most narrow to the most broad) and the design of activities to pursue those goals, ought to occur within the context of

- the organization's mission, vision, and plans;

- the needs and expectations of patients, staff, purchasers, and others;
- current knowledge about organizational and clinical activities;
- relevant historical data and external or comparative information; and
- availability of resources.

This examination of objectives may lead organization leaders to conclude that a new process is needed (or that an existing process needs to be redesigned).

Mission, Vision, and Plans

Throughout the organization, activities should serve the organization's mission (its prevailing purpose), its vision (how it sees itself in the future), and its plans (strategies for carrying out its mission and fulfilling its vision). An environmental assessment is one source of information used to establish mission, vision, and plans, and analyze whether current activities are useful and responsive in that context.

Needs and Expectations of Patients, Staff, and Others

In any health care organization, one goal is to understand the needs and expectations of patients/clients/residents and their families. These groups are the primary consumers of the health care organization's services, and meeting or exceeding their needs is critical to the organization's survival. (Their expectations are conscious desires related to the organization's services, whereas they may or may not be aware of their needs.) Once the needs and expectations are understood, the organization can decide how and to what extent they can be met.

Similarly, the staff of an organization are important "suppliers" of, and "customers" for, services the organization provides. Any consideration of organizational goals must take into account the needs and expectations of staff who will carry out and be affected by the process. Other important customers and suppliers to consider are purchasers, payers, accreditors, regulators, and the community as a whole.

Discussing the nine dimensions of performance in Chapter 1—

efficacy, appropriateness, availability, effectiveness, timeliness, safety, efficiency, continuity, and respect and caring—is an excellent way to elicit the needs and expectations of specific groups. Measures can then be put in place to determine whether performance fulfills those needs and expectations.

Current Knowledge about Organizational and Clinical Activities

An organization's goals—and the activities that pursue those goals—must reflect the best available knowledge about management and clinical activities. Management or support activities may include such processes as billing and scheduling. If, for example, an organization wants to change its scheduling practices, it should consider current practices within the organization and state-of-the-art practices. An organization can learn about state-of-the-art practices from expert sources both within and outside its walls; such sources include other similar health care organizations, nonhealth care organizations with similar processes, literature, professional societies, consultants, and others.

Likewise, expert knowledge of current practices—inside and outside the organization—is crucial in the design of any clinical activities. Such clinical knowledge can be captured in clinical algorithms, parameters of care, the scientific "literature," practice guidelines, standards of care, and others.

Several of the examples in this chapter and throughout this book show organizations using the knowledge of experts on particular subjects as a tool for successful design and improvement.

Relevant Data

Successful designs (as well as successful improvement efforts) require data. The importance of valid, reliable data, and effective use of those data cannot be overemphasized. For example, an organization would not decide to construct a new emergency department without knowledge about patient volume, staffing, equipment use, and so on. For redesign and other improvement efforts, information about patient outcomes is especially valuable; that information should encompass both performance within the organization (for example, aggregate data showing historical rates of specific outcomes for specific diagnoses) and information from reference databases. Information from reference databases—compiled by states, health care systems, payers, the Joint Commission, and others—can help organizations determine their goals for clinical outcomes. Use of aggregate data in performance improvement is described in more detail in Chapter 3 and elsewhere in this book.

Availability of Resources

In the current climate, health care organizations are painfully aware that their resources are limited. Every organization seeks ways to control costs and improve efficiency without sacrificing quality. In their short- and long-range planning, organizations face daunting decisions as they weigh their mission and vision against their resources. Organizations contemplating a new design effort will certainly weigh the availability of resources against the potential benefits—for patients and for the organization—of the new function or process to be designed. The ideal is to integrate quality planning and business planning. The visionary leader's dreams and the operations manager's pragmatism need to be reconciled with current resources.

II. WHAT AND HOW DO WE DESIGN?

As an organization identifies and weighs its goals, it must also examine the activities that will fulfill those goals. A productive way to view the activities of an organization is in terms of functions and processes. As described in Chapter 1, a function is a group of processes with a common goal, and a process is a series of linked, goal-directed activities. By focusing on functions and processes, an organization can design coordinated activities rather than isolated tasks. Activities are not performed for their own sake, but in service of a goal.

Therefore, when addressing what to design, we think in terms of functions and processes, in terms of the everyday work of health care organizations. Design of functions and processes occurs at many levels of generality or specificity. For example, "function" can refer to the entire health care organization as a complex system. Or "function" can refer to a multidisciplinary, cross-service activity such as patient assessment. "Process" can refer to the systematic way that nurses assess postoperative pain. Or "process" can refer to the specific steps for labelling specimens for transport from an extended care facility or the home to the laboratory. Or "process" can relate to how ambulatory patients are scheduled for clinic appointments or the organized way in which intakes for individuals with mental health problems are completed.

Any new process design must pay careful attention to interdependent activities, to the customer-supplier relationships inherent in the process. The design should facilitate the greatest efficiency in these relationships, coordinating and integrating the activities to produce desirable outcomes.

When deciding on a new process or function to design, the organization must carefully consider the

- organization's mission, vision, and plans;
- needs and expectations of patients, staff, and others;
- current knowledge about the process;
- relevant data; and
- available resources.

Ultimately, the decision weighs the benefits to patients and the organization against necessary resources.

To actually create a new design for patient care, management, or support processes, organizations will want to consider the following guidelines:

- *Design a systematic method to determine the process' effect on the organization's mission, vision, plans, customers, resources, and so forth.* Surveys, informal discussions, focus groups, and consensus techniques should be part of this process.
- *Base decisions on valid, reliable data.* Data are persuasive tools in determining how to design a process well, and are key to developing accurate design specifications and to assessing the effectiveness of the design.
- *Involve the right people.* Any design effort should include representatives of all groups who are responsible for, who

participate in, and who are affected by the process.

- *Obtain a variety of information on the subject.* Examine the literature, practices in other organizations, and advice of professional societies. Although each organization has its own experts, a view of other organizations' practices and experiences can help avoid mistakes and inspire creative thinking.

III. WHO CREATES THE DESIGN?

Organization leaders and managers are key players in the design process. The responsibility for overseeing design is a significant one. Leaders and managers must take an active role in setting priorities for design. Generally, managers are responsible for overseeing the design of processes within their areas; design of processes with a wider scope may be overseen by upper management or by a team of middle managers. Leaders must make sure the right people are involved in the effort and that these people have the necessary resources and expertise. Finally, leaders must make sure the right people are empowered, that is, their authority to make changes is commensurate with their responsibility for process improvements. Although regular feedback and contact with management is important, rigid control can stifle creativity.

The group that creates the process should include the people responsible for the process, the people who will carry out the process, and the people affected by the process. As appropriate, the members come from different departments, different disciplines, and different levels. When the group needs a perspective not offered by its representatives, it should get that perspective through interviews, through surveys, or by inviting new members into the work group.

IV. EXAMPLES OF DESIGN

————————————— *Automated Patient Record[1]* —————————————

Introduction

This example recounts the efforts of a 362-bed urban teaching hospital to automate its patient record. The project spans ap-

———

proximately 14 years, from the late 1970s to the present. The project's large timespan indicates that design work is not always a short-term, one-shot effort.

Design activities can involve multiple phases, each of which may include some measurement to assure that the project is proceeding as planned and, if not, appropriate modifications should be made. Note that one component of the cycle for improving performance does not have to be completed before another is begun.

Design work must be driven by explicit objectives, which in this example are defined by the hospital's senior management team. Note also that this design process is carried out by a multidisciplinary, multidepartmental team drawn from the areas most affected by the proposed change. The team seeks state-of-the-art knowledge, considers customer and staff input, and visits other hospitals that have gone through similar experiences en route to developing a multiyear phase-in plan for automating the whole record.

Example

The decision to investigate automating the medical record is based on several factors. Considering these factors, senior management sets the following objectives for an automated patient record:

- To help the hospital keep pace with the rapid changes in health care delivery;
- To improve patient care by improving accuracy and timeliness of the information used to manage patient care;
- To improve working conditions for staff;
- To improve data accuracy for a wide range of activities, from billing to quality improvement; and
- To improve efficiency throughout the hospital.

The hospital creates a team of representatives from all key departments and disciplines. This team is charged with analyzing the hospital's information management needs and comparing available systems with those needs.

The team conducts extensive surveys and other data collection to determine

- the needs an automated system must meet;

- the equipment and expertise that will be necessary;
- the systems available;
- the computer expertise in the organization;
- the attitudes of staff toward an automated record; and
- the attitudes of payers, purchasers, and patients toward an automated record.

For example, the team uses the average census, number of staff, usual volume of orders, typical amount of charting, and geographical constraints to determine the number of computer terminals each unit would need.

As part of its assessment of available systems, the team collects information about the state of the art in automated systems. The team also visits two hospitals currently using automated systems. These site visits provide vivid evidence of how such a system operates on a day-to-day basis; the team pays careful attention to anecdotes and data showing benefits and drawbacks.

The team systematically weighs the issues involved, comparing the capabilities of the systems being considered against the hospital's needs, the hospital personnel's capabilities, and the hospital's resources; considering the cost in the context of other hospital budgetary considerations; and comparing the findings of the site visits. The team is especially interested in a system that fulfills clinical information management needs, not just financial information needs. The team believes that such a system will help the hospital meet its future needs. (In the late 1970s, when this selection process was taking place, few automated hospital information systems were proficient in clinical areas; their strengths were the financial areas.) Based on these considerations, the team recommends a system to senior management. The recommendation is not a surprise because senior management has been kept apprised during the entire selection process.

The implementation plan (which the hospital calls "Stagecoach to Star Wars") defines specific stages. The underlying intention is for each component to be functioning well before the next is implemented. An overview of implementation follows:

1981-1983

- Finance system.
- Admission, discharge, and transfer system.
- Order entry for inpatient and outpatient areas and emergency department.

1983-1985

- Laboratory and radiology results.
- Physician use—to generate patient lists and retrieve diagnostic results.
- Nursing work lists and physician-to-nurse orders.
- Day surgery center/outpatient testing facility (implements all existing functions).

1985-1986

- Planning for nursing implementation.

1986

- All aspects of nursing documentation (assessments, notes, care plans, and others) automated on all units.

1987-1989

- Nursing acuity/patient classification system.
- Switchboard.

1990

- Physician sign-in and sign-out.

1991

- Respiratory therapy.
- Occupational therapy.
- Speech therapy.
- Dietary services.

As of 1991, two-thirds of the medical record is automated, with plans being formulated to automate the remainder.

At all phases, the team collects data and assesses the findings to determine the effect of the changes. Among the results are

- improved accreditation survey findings related to documentation and quality improvement;
- over 90% approval rating from nursing;
- reduced nursing turnover; and
- reduced rates of incomplete and delinquent records.

In addition, the state malpractice insurer has voiced its favorable impression of the system (after initial skepticism).

————————— *Emergency Department Patient Flow[2]* —————————

Introduction

The distinction between design and redesign work is not always clear, as this example illustrates. Clearly, the hospital had some existing mechanisms for managing patient flow in the emergency service. However, because the team that examined this important process started with no preconceptions, they thought of their work as design.

The label is not important. Rather, this example illustrates how routine measurement (in this case, of trauma care timeliness, patient volume, and acuity) can stimulate a re-examination of the hospital's mission, vision, and strategic plan, as reflected in one major service area. Note that the project team elicits opinions from patients, hospital colleagues, and outside experts. Design of a better process is aided by breaking the emergency department system into component parts, including clinical activities like triage and patient assessment and disposition and organizational activities like information flow, staffing, and security.

Example

On an ongoing basis, this hospital has been measuring certain processes involved in emergency care. These measures include several of the Joint Commission's recommended trauma indicators, including ones related to timeliness. The measurements, when assessed in comparison to the hospital's goals, lead the hospital to attempt to improve patient flow through the emergency department. However, several tested actions to

improve the existing process fail to result in desired performance. Because of the increased use of the emergency department, the hospital's mission to provide emergency care, and the
limited-scale attempts to improve patient flow were unsuccess-
ful, the hospital assembles a team to design the patient flow
through the emergency department.

The team includes representatives from administration, medical staff, nursing, human resources, facilities management, security, and clerical staff. Each member offers valuable expertise
from his or her area.

The design process includes establishing goals for the emergency department and ensuring that these goals reflect the
hospital's mission, strategic plans, and financial plans. These
goals draw on department standards of care and standards from
clinical literature and the state's reference database.

The process also includes further measurement and assessment of issues such as patient volume and patient acuity. The
study and design address processes such as triage, registration,
patient assessment, medical and nursing staffing, information
flow, ancillary services, medical staff coverage/response, patient
discharge, inpatient admission, direct admission, security, as
well as facility design as it pertains to these processes.
The team goes outside its own members for input; it consults
internal and external customers—patients, emergency physicians, nurses, laboratory personnel, information management
personnel, registration personnel, among others—as well as
facility design experts.

The team focuses on designing an ideal patient flow process,
rather than refining what the hospital already has. All team
members welcome the opportunity to make their long-standing
concerns known, and to ensure that the new design supports their
efforts to give patients the care they need.

Comments

Both of these examples encapsulate versions of how organizations
can successfully design a process. In both cases, the organizations select the process only after carefully considering the effect

on the organization's mission, vision, and plan, and on staff, patients, and other customers and suppliers. The organizations involve all the people important to the process. The teams collect data about needs and expectations, practices outside the organization, and resource implications. These data then form the basis for the design and the implementation plan.

Other examples in this book present more details about how organizations design processes.

V. SUMMARY POINTS

- *Why do we design?* Design requires setting objectives based on
  - the organization's mission, vision, and plans;
  - the needs and expectations of patients, staff, and others;
  - current knowledge about organizational and clinical activities;
  - information about performance and outcomes; and
  - availability of resources.
- *What and how do we design?*
  - Design focuses on functions and processes.
  - Successful designs are created by using a systematic method, basing decisions on data, involving the right people, and finding the best information.
- *Who creates the design?*
  - Leaders set priorities for design.
  - The process' owners, suppliers, and customers create the design, with experts as necessary.

REFERENCES

1. Miller C: A clinical case study: Moving toward an automated patient record. *Topics in Health Information Management* 13(4):30-35, 1993.

2. Greenberg L, Markin DA: Enhancing patient flow in the emergency department, *Leadership and Management in Emergency Nursing* 2 (6). Park Ridge, IL: Emergency Nurses Association, 1993.

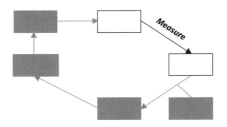

Chapter 3
MEASURE

No matter what process or function you want to examine—from mammography screening to fire safety education to the use of restraints to discharge planning to maintaining food temperature to provision of home parenteral nutrition to telephone coverage—you need data. Without data, a group can only exchange anecdotes, hunches, and impressions. These things are all worth considering; they should be heard, and they do have a place in an improvement effort. But to build an improvement effort on such "evidence" alone is insufficient. Thus, the goal of measurement is to provide data that objectively describe how a function or process is operating and what its results or outputs are.

Cycle for Improving Performance—Measure

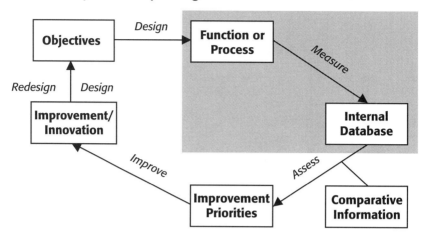

Figure 3-1. *This figure highlights the **measure** stage of the improvement cycle—the subject of this chapter.*

Measurement is by no means unfamiliar in health care. Organizations routinely measure response to therapy, equipment safety, test accuracy, staffing levels, costs...the list seems endless. In this chapter, we discuss how measurement works within the cycle for improving performance.

In today's environment, accountability is an especially pressing concern. Health care organizations are being compared to one another, and they must be prepared to demonstrate empirically, with data, that their care is efficacious, appropriate, available, timely, effective, safe, efficient, continuous, and respectful and caring. This requires organizations to quantify their performance with measures of patient health outcomes, satisfaction, and resource consumption. Every health care reform proposal includes requirements for measuring performance. For example, President Clinton's national Health Security Plan proposes a National Quality Management Program that includes an array of measurement activities, including developing quality and performance measures and setting national goals for performance on selected quality measures.[1]

To help health care organizations collect the data they need

Cycle for Improving Performance–Measurement Issues

Purpose and types of measurement
• Ongoing measurement
• Intensive measurement
• Measurement to determine improvement

Priorities for measurement
• Important functions (patient care and organizational)
• High-volume, high risk, and problem-prone functions/processes
• Functions/processes of special concern (to patients, staff, organizational mission)

Indicators
• Aggregate and sentinel event
• Process and outcome

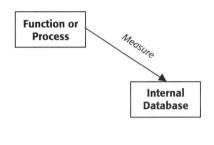

Figure 3-2. *These issues are addressed by organizations measuring performance as part of the cycle.*

to improve performance, this chapter answers the following core questions:

• Why do we measure?

• What do we measure?

• How do we measure?

• Who performs the measurement?

This information will guide organizations in achieving the result of measurement: a performance database. Figure 3-1, page 52 illustrates the place of measurement in the cycle for improving performance. Figure 3-2 shows some of the major considerations in performance measurement.

In addition, this chapter provides readers with specific examples of how organizations measure their performance, information about the Joint Commission's indicator measurement system, and a summary of key concepts.

For an even more detailed treatment of this subject, readers should consult two other Joint Commission books devoted to measurement: *The Measurement Mandate* and *Primer on Indicator Development and Application.*

I. WHY DO WE MEASURE?
THE PURPOSE OF MEASUREMENT

The last chapter described how to design a function or process, which is where the improvement cycle often begins. Once functions or processes are underway, an organization should collect data about its performance.

Measurement, in our present context, is the process by which we collect these data.[2] Measurement is not an end in itself, but rather a step that leads to assessment to transform data into information that helps answer such questions as: What is the level of performance? Are improvement actions necessary? What actions should be taken? Measurement is also the tool for determining whether improvement has occurred.

More specifically, one purpose of measurement is to provide a baseline when little objective evidence exists about a process. For example, a hospital committee for medication use may want to learn more about how physicians are using a drug recently added to the formulary, or staff on an adolescent psychiatric unit may want to know more about the use and effect of "time out" procedures. Measurement for this purpose may use specific indicators (such as a particular outcome or a particular step in a process) for ongoing data collection. Once assessed, these data can help staff determine when a process requires further attention, which could involve more intensive measurement and analysis. Data about costs, including costs of "dis-quality" (for example, the cost of repeat laboratory tests) may also be of significant interest to organization leaders and can be part of ongoing performance measurement.

Measurement is also important when a decision has been made to improve a process. As stated in the previous paragraph, a decision to improve a process can be based on measurement and assessment of the resulting data. For example, perhaps a target performance rate has not been met (such as a complication rate or length of stay related to coronary artery bypass grafts); perhaps a performance rate varies significantly from the rate during the previous year, varies between different shifts, or varies with statistical significance from the average; perhaps patient or staff feedback indicates dissatisfaction with or questions about performance. Such findings may cause an organization to focus on a given process to determine opportunities for improvement. Detailed measurement would then be necessary to gather data about exactly how the process performs and what factors affect that performance.

Finally, measurement is necessary to demonstrate the effect of an improvement action. Once you change a process, you will need some way to determine whether performance improves. If, for instance, a managed care organization institutes a new procedure to encourage well-baby care, the organization will not only need a baseline rate of current visits for well-baby care, but will need to continue measuring that rate after the new procedure is adopted to make sure improvement occurs. Measurement is also necessary to demonstrate that key processes (for example, delivery of stat medications) are in control. For example, once a process has been stabilized at an acceptable level of performance, measures may be taken periodically to verify that the improvement has been sustained.

The result of measurement is an organization-specific performance database. This database may contain information about process performance, outcomes, satisfaction, cost, and judgments about quality and value.

II. WHAT DO WE MEASURE? PRIORITIES FOR MEASUREMENT

A health care organization cannot constantly measure everything. Its activities are too diverse and its resources are limited. Therefore, the organization's leaders must find the most productive way to measure the most important processes in the organization. One way to measure a wide range of processes is to measure certain outcomes and/or certain parts of a process that can potentially identify larger performance issues. This is referred to as "screening." For example, a home care agency could measure the rate of interruptions in infusion therapy to find potential opportunities to improve that process. For another example, a chemical dependency program can monitor the recidivism rate to help determine the effectiveness of certain types of treatment. When performance rates in these areas show significant variation or do not achieve

Matrix Used to Determine Key Processes

Department: 3 West   ● Heavy   ◉ Moderate   ○ Slight

	Indicators	Impact	Process 1	Process 2	Process 3
Physician	Available time	●	MD rounds update	Chart procedure	Procedure assist
	Scheduling	○	Requisition process		
	Nurses	●	MD rounds update	Procedure assist	Complication notification
	Timely reports	◉	Filing	Abnormal result notification	Requisition process
	Consultants accessible	○	Order notification		
	Equipment				
Patient	Clinical outcome	●	Acute MI	Bronchitis	Heart failure
	Response TLC	●	Pain medication	Nourishment	Call light response
	Nurses	●	Patient condition inform	Nurse skills assessment & CE	Complaint notification
	Living arrangement	◉	Complaint notification	Discharge cleaning	Diet order
	Admission	○	Discharge cleaning		
	Discharge	●	Discharge notification	Discharge instructions	Transport

Figure 3-3. *This matrix is used to determine and rank the processes that support customer expectations.* **Source:** *West Paces Medical Center, Atlanta. Used with permission.*

targets, more detailed measurement (and assessment) can be initiated.

Organizations must not only decide how to conduct ongoing measurement, but must decide which processes to measure. Leaders will want to devote much attention to this matter, carefully weighing the organization's processes in terms of its mission, vision, and resources, in addition to provider, patient, community, purchaser, and payer concerns.

Figure 3-3 shows one medical center's method for identifying important processes to measure. In this method, the hospital surveys its major "customers"—patients, physicians, employees, and payers—regarding the qualities they most desire in the hospital. These qualities (called "indicators" in this example) are placed on a matrix. Each customer group then identifies processes that support these qualities and determines their impact. The results help identify the most important processes to measure, assess, and improve.

Other important factors when choosing processes to continuously measure are any standards or requirements from regulating or accrediting bodies, including the Joint Commission. In its *Accreditation Manual for Hospitals*, for example, the Joint Commission targets a number of important functions, each of which must be the subject of ongoing measurement (see Table 1-3 from Chapter 1, page 20). This list of functions is worth considering not only because it forms part of the Joint Commission's standards, but also because it offers a valuable frame of reference for an acute care facility that is attempting to organize its measurement activities. These functions are intentionally broad; the standards allow considerable flexibility for measurement within each function.

For hospitals, the 1995 standards address the following important functions:

- *Care of the Patient Functions*
  - Patient rights and organizational ethics;
  - Assessment of patients;
  - Care of patients (including care planning, anesthesia care, medication use, nutritional care, operative and other invasive procedures, rehabilitation, and special treatment procedures;
  - Education; and
  - Continuum of care, including entry to setting or service, continuity, coordination, and discharge planning;
- *Organizational Functions*
  - Leadership;
  - Management of information;
  - Management of human resources;
  - Management of the environment of care;
  - Surveillance, prevention, and control of infection; and
  - Improving organizational performance.

The standards also identify certain important sources of data for measuring performance that a hospital should use:

- Staff views about the organization's performance and opportunities for improvement;
- Autopsy results;
- Risk management activities; and
- Quality control activities in at least clinical laboratory, diagnostic radiology, dietetic, nuclear medicine, and radiation oncology services.

Finally, measurement should also provide information about appropriateness of admissions and continued hospitalization (for example, utilization review).

Within the functions identified above, organizations must select specific processes to measure. The processes chosen should be those that

- affect a large percentage of patients; and/or
- place patients at serious risk if not performed well, or performed when not indicated, or not performed when indicated; and/or
- have been or are likely to be problem prone.

Organizations will also want to include customer reports, including customer satisfaction in its measurement. Customer feedback (for example, satisfaction surveys of patients and staff) can help an organization determine what process needs attention, can help identify a process' weaknesses and strengths, and can help measure improvement once changes have been made. This framework for improving performance directs attention to patients—the ultimate focus of health care. Therefore, it is logical for organizations to measure patient satisfaction with outcomes, with parts of the care process, and with dimensions of performance such as respect and caring, and to integrate this information into the organizationwide effort to improve performance.

III. HOW DO WE MEASURE? TYPES AND TOOLS OF MEASUREMENT

As mentioned earlier, health care organizations will carry out two basic types of measurement:

- Ongoing measurement about selected important processes; and

- Measurement about priority issues chosen for improvement.

The first type involves ongoing data collection about selected outcomes or aspects of the process. The second type of measurement is part of a more intensive assessment-and-improvement effort (which may have been initiated based on the results of ongoing measurement, including patient/staff feedback).

For example, a hospital may continuously collect data regarding unplanned admission to an ICU unit within one day after a procedure involving anesthesia. If that rate shows excessive variability or unacceptable performance levels, further assessment should be initiated. That assessment would entail more frequent, detailed data collection addressing issues such as types of procedures performed, patient risk factors, types of anesthesia, practitioners involved, and so on. For example, if an improvement is subsequently made in the postanesthesia care process, outcomes should be tracked closely to determine the effect of the change.

Such measurement is based on indicators that capture the specific data to be collected. Measurement also requires tools to collect and display the data. The following sections offer an overview of indicator use. For a more comprehensive treatment of indicator use, refer to *The Measurement Mandate* and *Primer on Indicator Development and Application*, available from the Joint Commission. The information on indicators that follows is drawn from those sources.[2,3]

Definition of Indicator

An indicator is a valid and reliable quantitative process or outcome measure related to one or more dimensions of performance, such as effectiveness and appropriateness. Much information is contained in that short definition. To fully understand that definition, we will break it into its key components (see Table 3-1, page 60).

Quantitative measure. Quantitative data are expressed in specific measurement units. These data alone do not express any judgment or conclusion about the process being measured. They provide specific, objective information requiring further analysis and interpretation.

An Indicator is

- **Quantitative**—expressed in units of measurement

- **Valid**—identifies events that merit review

- **Reliable**—accurately and completely identifies occurrences

- **A measure of outcome**—the results of performance—*or process*—a goal-directed series of activities.

Table 3-1. *Indicator Defined. An indicator is a valid and reliable quantitative process or outcome measure related to one or more dimensions of performance, such as effectiveness and appropriateness.*

Reliable and valid. An indicator is reliable if different observers (or the same observer on multiple occasions) obtain the same measurement for the same event. An indicator is valid if that measurement identifies an opportunity for improving performance (or identifies a phenomenon that merits further review, which is a step toward identifying an improvement opportunity).

Process or outcome. Indicators specify either a specific part of the process being measured or an outcome of that process. Outcome measurement is necessary to learn results, and process measurement is necessary to learn what caused those results. For example, the outcomes of many clinical processes may not be evident or measurable at discharge or they may vary considerably due to patient-specific factors. It is therefore more prudent to measure the processes that most profoundly influence the anticipated outcome as surrogate measures of the outcome.

An example of an outcome indicator is "Intrahospital mortality of patients undergoing isolated coronary artery bypass graft procedures," whereas an example of a process indicator is, "Trauma patients with prehospital emergency medical services scene time greater than 20 minutes."

With these concepts in mind, we can further describe indicators by reviewing their types.

Types of Indicators

The two broadest types of indicators are sentinel event indicators and aggregate data indicators. A sentinel event indicator identifies an individual event or phenomenon that is significant enough to trigger further investigation each time it occurs. Most sentinel events are undesirable and occur infrequently. The following are two examples of sentinel events in an acute-care setting:

- Patients developing a peripheral neurological deficit within two postprocedure days of procedures involving anesthesia administration; and
- Maternal death.

Such indicators are well known in risk management. They must be identified to assure that each event is promptly evaluated to prevent future occurrences. Although sentinel event indicators are useful to help assure patient safety, they are less useful in measuring the overall level of performance in an organization. Even when extremes of performance are removed, the mean remains basically the same.

An aggregate data indicator, in contrast, quantifies a process or outcome related to many cases. Unlike sentinel events, an event identified by an aggregate data indicator may occur frequently. Aggregate data indicators are divided into two groups: rate-based indicators and continuous-variable indicators.

Rate-based indicators. Some aggregate data indicators are expressed as rates. Sometimes that rate is a proportion, as in the three examples that follow:

$$\frac{\text{patients receiving cesarean sections}}{\text{all patients who deliver}}$$

$$\frac{\text{trauma patients with prehospital emergency medical services}}{\text{scene time greater than 20 minutes}}{\text{all trauma patients receiving prehospital emergency medical services}}$$

$$\frac{\text{mental health outpatients for whom more than two weeks elapse}}{\text{between referral and initiation of therapy}}{\text{all patients referred to the facility}}$$

A proportion shows the number of occurrences compared to the entire group within which the occurrence could take place.

The rate can also be expressed as a ratio—in which the occurrences identified are compared with a different (but related) phenomenon. For example,

$$\frac{\text{patients with central line infections}}{\text{central line days}}$$

Continuous variable indicators. This type of aggregate data indicator measures how performance falls along a continuous scale. For example, a continuous variable indicator might show the precise weight in pounds of an individual receiving total parenteral nutrition. Or, consider the example above concerning emergency medical services scene time for trauma patients. The rate-based indicator measures whether the scene time is or is not greater than 20 minutes. A continuous variable indicator, in contrast, would measure the specific scene time, thus offering more precise information.

Those designing the measurement activities must consider the process being measured, the goals of measurement, and the available data to choose the best type or types of indicators. (Table 3-2, page 63, summarizes the different types of indicators; the examples section of this chapter provides more illustrations of how indicators are used to measure performance.)

Using Indicators

When selecting or developing a measurement system, staff should consider these two important tips to assure a balanced system:

- Use different types of measures (for example, measures of process and outcome, sentinel event and aggregate data indicators); and
- Use measures sensitive to various dimensions of performance.

By selecting different types of measures, you will be more likely to capture data that illuminate various aspects of the process. Similarly, by using indicators that address the various dimensions of performance, you will help assure that measure-

Aggregate data indicator: A performance measure based on collection and aggregation of data about many events or phenomena. The events or phenomena may be desirable or undesirable, and the data may be reported as a continuous variable or as a discrete variable (or rate).

Continous variable indicator: An aggregate data indicator in which the value of each measurement can fall anywhere along a continuous scale (for example, the precise weight in pounds of an individual receiving parenteral nutrition).

Rate-based (or discrete variable) indicator: An aggregate data indicator in which the value of each measurement is expressed as a proportion or as a ratio. In a proportion, the numerator is expressed as a subset of the denominator (for example, patients with cesarean sections over all patients who deliver). In a ratio, the numerator and denominator measure different phenomena (for example, the number of patients with central lines who develop infections over central line days).

Sentinel event indicator: A performance measure that identifies an individual event or phenomenon that always triggers further analysis and investigation and that usually occurs infrequently and is undesirable in nature.

Table 3-2. *Types of Indicators*

ment does not ignore important aspects of the process and its performance.

You will recall that, in Chapter 1, we discussed the various dimensions of performance:

- Efficacy;
- Appropriateness;
- Availability;
- Effectiveness;
- Timeliness;
- Safety;
- Efficiency;
- Continuity; and
- Respect and caring.

No one of these dimensions eclipses the others; all are essential ingredients for an organization pursuing excellence in performance. And these dimensions do not exist independently;

The Quality Cube

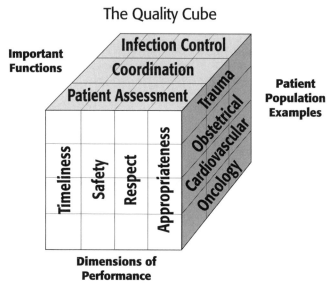

Figure 3-4. *This figure illustrates the connection between the dimensions of performance, important functions, and patient population types (choosing just a few examples of each).*

for example, improved availability of a service may influence its timeliness. For each function or process being measured, you should consider the relevant dimensions of performance and should tailor indicators to address them.

The cube in Figure 3-4 illustrates how important *functions, patient populations* (for example, DRGs, patients receiving specified procedures), and *dimensions of performance* intersect. Measurement may initially arise from any of these three factors (for example, from a function such as coordination of care, from a patient population such as trauma patients, or from a dimension of performance, such as safety). To determine what measures will be most useful, an organization can first look at the initial factor and then ascertain which of the remaining two factors are most relevant. For example, if a hospital is measuring care provided to trauma patients, it would probably focus on timeliness (a dimension of performance) of patient assessment (an important function). The measurement effort for this patient population is less likely to focus on, for example, whether patient education (important function) is delivered with respect and caring (dimension of performance).

IV. WHO PERFORMS THE MEASUREMENT?

Deciding who will measure performance is closely linked to the purposes and types of measurement. In other words, the people who select and design the measurement activities and the people who collect the data will differ depending on the goals of the measurement. The following paragraphs give a general idea of who may be responsible for various aspects and types of measurement.

Ongoing Screening to Collect Information About a Process

Health care organizations have various experts who should help design the ongoing measurement activities. These include experts in information management, quality improvement, and each function to be measured. The organization's leaders must at least review and approve the design of ongoing measurement.

The people who actually collect data from ongoing measurement will vary widely depending on the specific organization, the function being measured, and the measurement process. Information management professionals and those actually carrying out the process being measured will be key players in data collection. Organizations should make every effort to coordinate ongoing measurement with data collection already taking place as part of everyday activities.

Measurement for a Specific Improvement Effort

When an organization has decided to improve a particular process—from reporting adverse drug reactions to educating patients about home medical equipment—it may empower a specific group to study the process and recommend changes. Sometimes this group will be an existing working team; in other cases, especially when a process crosses department/service lines, a special team may be formed from among the process' owners, suppliers, and customers. This study will require measurement that is more detailed than routine screening. This team or workgroup, composed of experts in the process studied, will usually be responsible for designing and carrying out the measurement necessary to capture information about how the process performs. After making changes to improve the process, this group will usually continue applying some or all of its measures to determine whether the change has had the desired effect.

V. THE JOINT COMMISSION'S INDICATOR MEASUREMENT SYSTEM[4]

Measurement is fundamental to any accrediting body, including the Joint Commission. Historically, the Joint Commission has measured the performance of health care organizations through triennial, on-site evaluations of compliance with standards that, for the most part, addressed an organization's structures and processes, rather than outcomes. In 1986, the Joint Commission embarked on a major research-and-development initiative, the Agenda for Change, to create an evaluation system that could be used not only by the Joint Commission, but by others as well. The evaluation system would continue to include measures of standards compliance, but the standards would be focused on the organization's *actual performance* rather than on its *capability* to provide care.

The Agenda for Change project has three major components:

- Refocusing standards to address important clinical, managerial, support, and governance functions;
- Improving the survey process to address performance of these important functions; and
- Developing the capability to continuously monitor organizational performance using reliable and valid performance measures and an automated database.
- The third component of this initiative has coalesced into an *indicator measurement system* (IMSystem). The research and development of this system represent a significant advance in the ability to measure health care organizations' performance.

The IMSystem involves continuous collection of performance information related to specific indicators. This information can be used by health care organizations to improve performance, by the Joint Commission to evaluate health care organizations, and by other interested users (such as purchasers and payers) to make decisions about health care.

The IMSystem will be introduced in stages to organizations seeking accreditation. At first, participation will be voluntary, and the system will consist of ten indicators. Later, more indicators will be introduced, and participation will become a required component of the accreditation process.

Indicators Included

Indicators demonstrating sufficient relevance, reliability, and validity are eligible for the IMSystem. Of those indicators, a limited number will be in use at any given time. In 1994, the system includes ten indicators focusing on obstetrical and perioperative care.

(Table 3-3, page 68-69, lists the ten indicators approved for 1994. Appendix C also lists Joint Commission indicators currently being tested for validity and reliability, along with indicators offered for hospital internal use.)

In 1995, approximately ten more indicators will be added. These indicators will measure performance in trauma, oncology, and cardiovascular care. In 1996, indicators related to the functions of medication use and infection control will be included.

The IMSystem database will include data elements and assigned indicator categories at the patient level. More specifically, every patient record will include values for the necessary data elements, as well as a category assignment of that patient for each indicator in the system (for example, "patient experienced indicator #1," "patient is not in the population of interest for indicator #7," and so on). Receipt of both the data elements and indicator category assignments at the patient level is necessary to ensure that complete data are submitted and to maintain consistency across participating hospitals. The accuracy of comparative reports generated from the database depends on the data's accuracy, completeness, and consistency (reliability).

VI. EXAMPLES OF PERFORMANCE MEASUREMENT

This section presents various examples of how health care organizations measure performance. The examples illustrate the three purposes for measurement:

- Ongoing measurement to monitor a process;

Performance Measures—1994

1. **Numerator:** Patients developing a central nervous system (CNS) complication within two postprocedure days of procedures involving anesthesia* administration.

   Denominator: All patients undergoing surgical procedures involving anesthesia administration and having an inpatient stay.

2. **Numerator:** Patients developing a peripheral neurologic deficit within two postprocedure days of procedures involving anesthesia administration.

   Denominator: All patients undergoing surgical procedures involving anesthesia administration and having an inpatient stay.

3. **Numerator:** Patients developing an acute myocardial infarction (AMI) within two postprocedure days of procedures involving anesthesia administration.

   Denominator: All patients undergoing surgical procedures involving anesthesia administration and having an inpatient stay.

4. **Numerator:** Patients with a cardiac arrest within two postprocedure days of procedures involving anesthesia administration.

   Denominator: All patients undergoing surgical procedures involving anesthesia administration and having an inpatient stay.

5. **Numerator:** Intrahospital mortality of patients within two postprocedure days of procedures involving anesthesia administration.

   Denominator: All patients undergoing surgical procedures involving anesthesia administration and having an inpatient stay.

6. **Numerator:** Patients delivered by cesarean section.
   Denominator: All deliveries.

7. **Numerator:** Patients with vaginal birth after cesarean section (VBAC).
   Denominator: Patients delivered with a history of previous cesarean section.

8. **Numerator:** Live-born infants with a birthweight less than 2,500 grams.
   Denominator: All live births.

9. **Numerator:** Live-born infants with a birthweight greater than or equal to 2,500 grams, who have at least one of the following: an Apgar score of less than 4 at five minutes, a requirement for admission to the neonatal intensive care unit (NICU) within one day of delivery for greater than 24 hours, a clinically apparent seizure or significant birth trauma

Table 3-3. *Approved Indicators for 1994—continued on page 69.*

Performance Measures—1994 (continued)

Denominator: All live-born infants with a birthweight greater than or equal to 2,500 grams.

10. **Numerator:** Live-born infants with a birthweight greater than 1,000 grams and less than 2,500 grams who have an Apgar score of less than 4 at five minutes

   Denominator: All live-born infants with a birthweight greater than 1,000 grams and less than 2,500 grams

* For the indicators related to anesthesia care, the population of interest includes all patients undergoing surgical procedures involving anesthesia.

   Anesthesia is defined as the administration (in any setting, for any purpose, by any route) of general, spinal, or other major regional anesthesia or sedation (with or without analgesia) for which there is a reasonable expectation that, in the manner used, the sedation/analgesia will result in the loss of protective reflexes for a significant percentage of a group of patients.

Table 3-3. *Approved Indicators for 1994—continued from previous page.*

- Intensive measurement as part of an improvement effort; and
- Measurement to determine the effect of an improvement effort.

The examples are designed to provide a range of approaches to ongoing measurement; no one approach is the best for every organization, and none are specifically required by Joint Commission standards. Rather than creating hypothetical examples that follow unrealistic procedures, these are adapted from actual practices at various hospitals. The goal is diversity: to show the many possibilities for measuring performance.

Ongoing Measurement

These examples show how organizations obtain initial information about a process. The first example is the most broad: it summarizes a hospital system's process for continuously measuring patient outcomes for a wide range of diagnoses. The other examples are more focused, showing how organizations, having identified a particular process to measure, collect information about how that process is performing.

─────── *Patient outcomes in a multihospital system.*[5] ───────

Introduction

Just as functions or processes can be thought of broadly or narrowly, measurement can also be quite broad at times and very focused at other times. This example illustrates measurement at a high level—across all institutions in a multihospital system—of global outcomes such as length of stay and mortality.

Example

In this system, hospitals annually provide patient discharge abstracts to the system headquarters. These abstracts, which are sent on computer tape, are based on the Universal Hospital Discharge Data Set. This information is then sent to a consultant. The consultant

- rates each discharge according to severity of illness;
- retrieves information about
  - hospital admission patterns (according to major disease category and DRG),
  - patient characteristics (comorbidities, stage of illness), and
  - patient outcomes (satisfactory outcomes, short length of stay, long length of stay, potentially avoidable complications, and death);
- compares data in these areas with those from selected comparison groups; and
- for all DRGs, identifies statistically significant differences between individual hospitals and comparison groups.

The results are shared with individual hospitals in an educational—not a punitive—context. Individual hospitals report to headquarters about follow-up assessment of the findings.

───────── *Medication administration.*[6] ─────────

Introduction

Measurement may be applied to a process that is important for several reasons: because it puts patients at risk if done incorrectly, because it is performed frequently, and/or because it has been problematic in the past. This example shows how one hospital collected data about medication errors, an intermediate outcome in the medication administration process.

Example

Having identified medication administration as a high-volume, high-risk, and problem-prone process, one hospital unit sets out to design a continuous measurement tool for that process. First, a multidisciplinary group creates a flowchart to help understand the process and key points that could lead to medication errors (see Figure 3-5, page 72). Next, the group creates a tracking tool for medication errors. This tool corresponds to the flowchart and provides information that could be helpful in determining the nature and cause of the error (see Figure 3-6, page 73). By linking the data-collection instrument to the flowchart, the group system-izes information about outcomes (medication errors) to help the hospital understand the process of medication administration.

Postoperative cardiac care.[7]

Introduction

Indicators are useful measurement tools when they encourage a search for underlying causes or for explanations of data that have been collected. Such is the case in the following example. Three different types of indicators (a process measure, an outcome mea-sure, and a financial measure) lead to an examination of a cardiac care system.

Example

Several of the indicators continuously measured at this hospital provide information related to postoperative cardiac care. These include

- waiting time for, and cancellations of, cardiac surgery;
- postoperative length of stay (eight days is the goal); and
- charge per case.

   Findings related to these indicators suggest an opportunity to improve postoperative care processes: excessive waiting times

Medication Order, Delivery, and Administration Process Flowchart

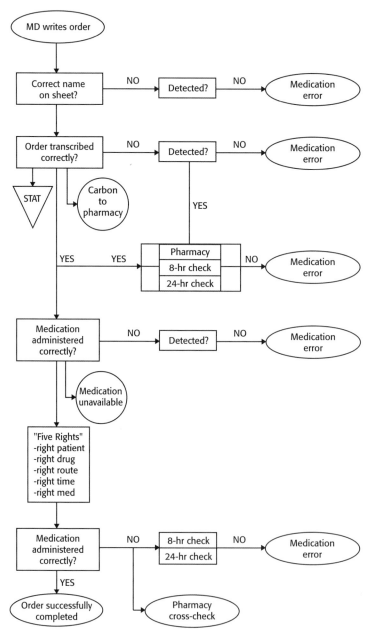

Figure 3-5. *This flowchart is used to detect steps in the medication process that may lead to errors. The tracking form in Figure 3-6 is linked to this chart.*
Source: *Bechtel GA et al: A continuous quality improvement approach to medication administration.* Journal of Nursing Care Quality *7 (3): 30, April 1993. Used with permission.*

Medication Order, Delivery, and Administration Process

Medication Administration Tracking Form

Day	Time	Room	Staff member	Acuity points	Nature	Cause	Effect	PTWY	Drug/ route	Comments

Nature	Cause	Effect
1 = Transciption	1 = Omission	1 = None noted
2 = Carelessness	2 = Wrong dose	2 = Minimum change
3 = Documentation	3 = Wrong med	3 = Moderate change
4 = _____	4 = Wrong time	4 = Significant change
	5 = Wrong client	5 = Critical incident
	6 = Wrong mode	6 = Significant cost
	7 = Delayed stat	7 = _____
	8 = _____	

Figure 3-6. *The team develops this form to collect and sort data related to medication errors. The "cause" section is derived from the flowchart in Figure 3-5.* **Source:** *Bechtel GA et al: A continuous quality improvement approach to medication administration.* Journal of Nursing Care Quality *7 (3): 30, April 1993. Used with permission.*

and cancellations are often traced to an inadequate number of surgical intensive care unit beds, post op lengths of stay regularly exceed the goal of eight days, and payers indicate that per-patient charges are higher than those in other institutions.

Informal communication also indicates a possible opportunity for improvement. Some newly hired staff mention different practice patterns in their previous hospitals—specifically, extubation within 5 to 10 hours post-op rather than this hospital's current 18 to 20 hours.

As a result of these findings, more detailed measurement and assessment are initiated.

———————————— *Medication use.*[8] ————————————

Introduction

The following example shows how indicators can be drawn from
existing data sources. It is not necessary to start from scratch when
selecting measures for continuous monitoring, because many of the
data elements will have already been collected for other purposes.
This hospital has designated two of its pharmacists as "opportu-
nity-for-improvement" staff. As "process owners" (that is, those
persons closest to the work), their job duties include data retrieval.

Example

Medication use is a key patient care function at any hospital. To
continuously monitor this function, one hospital considers the
existing data sources, the important events that can be seen in
these sources, and the value to patients of monitoring these events.
Table 3-4, page 75, shows the results of this effort. Data sources
include adverse drug reaction reports, concurrent drug usage
evaluation, and computer summaries of doses outside preset
ranges. Related events include dispensing errors, drug interactions,
and overrides of warnings related to doses outside the preset limits.
Based on this information, the pharmacy quality improvement
committee drafts indicators, which are then reviewed by all pharmacists and technicians. Data for the indicators are collected by
the department's two "opportunity" pharmacists.

INTENSIVE MEASUREMENT

Once a process is targeted, organizations collect detailed data
about that process as a stepping stone to improvement. The following examples illustrate how health care organizations conduct
this intensive measurement.

——— *Patient recovery following total joint replacement.*[9] ———

Introduction

In the following example, comparative data (about length of stay)
and financial data (showing a loss) for patients in DRG 209 (major joint replacement) created concern among staff in the joint
replacement "product line." A team organized and drew up a pro-

Data Used for Outcome Assessment and their Value to the Patient

Data source	Factors to be reviewed	Value to the patient
Medication error reports	• Order entry errors • Dispensing errors	• Medication error reporting is required by the Joint Commission for medical staff QI; use by the pharmacy is a bonus. Order entry errors and dispensing errors were previously monitored by sampling; use of medication error reports has consistently given higher numbers. Sampling has been discontinued. Corrective action is taken as trends are identified or as significant isolated events signal future problems.
ADR reports	• Order entry errors • Dispensing errors • Dispensing a medication to which the patient is allergic • Drug interactions • Dispensing medications with preservatives to neonates	• Adverse drug reaction reporting is required by the Joint Commission for medical staff QI; use by the pharmacy is a bonus. Identification of pharmacy's involvement in adverse drug reactions offers the opportunity to improve departmental systems and professional competency.
Pharmacist intervention log	• RPh response to nonformulatory orders • RPh response to inappropriate orders: dose/drug/route/ regimen/duration/ contraindications • RPh participation in concurrent drug usage evaluations	• The dose, route, regimen, duration, and contraindications (stated allergies) for all drugs are monitored concurrently at order entry. Use the intervention log to document contact with physicians and actions taken. From the pharmacy QI perspective, this documentation is used to monitor clinical decisions of the pharmacists. This monitoring provides a safety net at a time when patient outcome can still be affected. From the medical staff QI perspective, the physicians' responses to the pharmacists' interventions are reviewed.
Computer summaries	• Overrides of warnings of doses outside pre-set ranges • Overrides of drug interaction warnings	• Concurrently (generally within 24 hours) review dose and drug interaction overrides to intercept significant therapeutic misadventures.
•Drug information requests	• Accuracy of RPh responses	• Concurrently (generally within 24 hours) review responses to correct mistakes.
•Lab drug level summaries	• Drug levels outside therapeutic range	• Concurrently (generally within 24 hours) review drug therapy and contact physicians as necessary to recommend therapy change.

***Table 3-4.** **Source:** Powers SM: How to assemble a patient-centered pharmacy QI program,* Topics in Hospital Pharmacy Management *13 (2): 46-54, 1993. Used with permission.*

cess description in the form of a critical pathway that then guided intensive data collection about a limited number of cases.

Example

Continuous data collection at one hospital shows that length of stay for DRG 209 is three days more than that of other area hospitals. Additional data on practice patterns for prosthesis use note inappropriate variation. Also, cost data show an annual loss of $100,000 for these procedures. These findings trigger an intensive measurement, assessment, and improvement effort.

The team formed to study total joint replacements decides to narrow its focus to the most frequent of these procedures: total hip replacement. To fully understand the process involved in total hip replacement, the team creates a "critical pathway": a day-by-day, department-by-department delineation of the patient care process. The team uses this process to collect data from 25 cases. From these data, the following findings warrant further attention:

- Patients stayed in bed as long as 22 hours a day;
- Many patients received one physical therapy session a day (rather than the desired two to three); and
- For some patients, the social work assessment was delayed.

The team's next step is to determine the root causes for these findings.

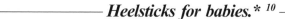

Heelsticks for babies. * [10]

Introduction

Sentinel events, such as an avoidable patient injury, often necessitate follow-up data colection. This is the case with the following example concerning bruised babies and the subsequent decision to expand measurement to include more descriptive data. These data help to determine root causes for heelstick bruises.

Example

After two babies are badly bruised, nursing and clinical laboratory managers at this hospital decide to assess the heelstick process for babies. A multidisciplinary team is formed. Among

---

* This example is adapted from the experiences of University Hospital in Denver.

the team's early activities are the identification of the process'
customers and suppliers and the creation of a flowchart to better
understand the process. The team also collects data about heelsticks on all babies in the NCU for one month. The data include

- who performs the heelstick;
- supplies used;
- time of each draw;
- blood tests done;
- number of resticks; and
- level of trauma.

These data are used to uncover the root causes for bruising
and to study the use patterns.

MEASUREMENT TO DETERMINE EFFECT OF ACTIONS

These examples show how organizations determine if actions to
improve care have the desired effect over time.

Heelsticks.[10]

Example

Continuing with the example above, the laboratory and nursing
team create four outcome indicators to continuously measure
performance of heelsticks on babies. These indicators do not
provide the kind of detailed information collected as part of the
intensive assessment; rather, they provide baseline data against
which to judge performance once actions are taken to improve the
process. These indicators also will allow continued measurement to
assure improvement is maintained and will create a performance
database. The four indicators are

- absence of bruises on legs and ankles (associated with
  heelsticks);
- absence of bruises on heels in puncture areas;
- presence of punctures in recommended draw areas; and
- fewer than five punctures per day (unless medically indicated).

Figure 3-7, page 78, shows run charts that illustrate findings for each indicator over 29 months.

Heelstick Process—Run Charts for Four Indicators

The four graphs show the percentage of babies with leg or ankle bruising, the percentage with heel bruising, the percentage with punctures in the recommended area, and the percentage who had fewer than five punctures per day. The drop in process performance at month 17 occurred when stricter evaluation criteria were applied.

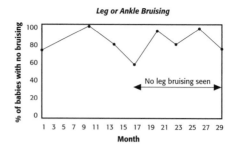

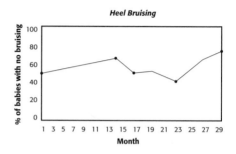

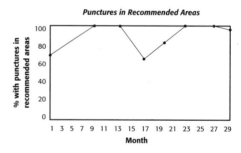

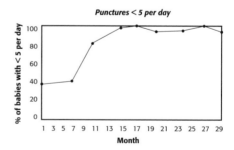

Figure 3-7. *Each run chart documents performance related to one indicator chosen to measure the heelstick process before and after the improvement actions.*
Source: *Romfh PC et al: Babies provide focus for quality improvement team.* Clinical Laboratory Management Review, *Mar/Apr 1993, p 151. Copyright Clinical Laboratory Management Association. Used with permission.*

———— *Emergency department admission times.*[11] ————

Introduction

When time is of the essence, measures should be put in place to answer the question, "How long does it take to measure whatever it is you want to measure?" In this example, time intervals are treated as intermediate outcomes that reflect the efficiency of antecedent processes.

Example

In this hospital, a team has been formed to study and improve time from triage to departure from the emergency department (and inpatient admission). Early in its efforts, the team identifies two continuous variable indicators:

- The interval between the time a patient was seen at the emergency department triage desk to the time a decision was made to admit the patient (T1-T2); and

- The interval between the time a decision was made to admit the patient to the time the patient left the emergency department en route to an inpatient unit (T2-T3).

These indicators allow continuous measurement of the process. They create a baseline against which the effects of improvement actions can be seen. The run chart in Figure 3-8, page 80, shows performance related to these indicators starting before the improvement interventions and continuing 16 months after.

VII. SUMMARY POINTS

- *Why do we measure?*
  - To gain information about performance on an ongoing basis.
  - To gain detailed information about a process chosen for assessment and improvement.
  - To determine the effect of improvement actions.
- What do we measure?
  - Selected high-volume, high-risk, and/or problem-prone processes (on an ongoing basis).
  - Selected processes as indicated by ongoing measurement or other feedback.

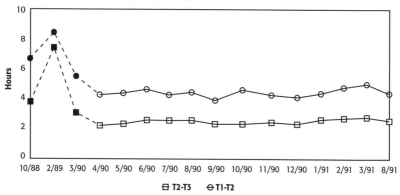

Figure 3-8. *The team uses this run chart to measure and assess performance before and after the process changes. T1-T2 is the interval between the time a patient was seen at the emergency department triage desk to the time a decision was made to admit the patient; T2-T3 is the interval between the time a decision was made to admit the patient to the time the patient left the emergency depart-ment en route to an inpatient unit. Open symbols are pre-intervention; solid symbols are post-intervention.* **Source:** *Goldmann DA et al: Hospital-based continuous quality improvement: a realistic appraisal.* Clinical Performance and Quality Health Care *1(2): 75, 1993. Used with permission.*

- Customer satisfaction.
- *How do we measure?*
    - With indicators of process or outcome. Indicators can identify sentinel events or can show aggregate performance.
- *Who performs the measurement?*
    - Leaders decide what to measure on an ongoing basis.
    - Work groups or other teams measure processes chosen for intensive assessment and improvement.
- *The product of measurement is a performance database.*
    - The database provides aggregate information about pro-cess performance, outcomes, satisfaction, cost, and judgments about quality.
- *The Joint Commission's IMSystem collects performance data from accredited organizations.*
    - As of 1994, the IMSystem consists of ten indicators hospi-tals can use on a voluntary basis.
    - The system will later become part of the accreditation process, at which time participation will be mandatory.

REFERENCES

1. The White House Domestic Policy Council: *The President's Health Security Plan.* New York: Times Books, 1993, pp 112-113.

2. Joint Commission on Accreditation of Healthcare Organizations: *The Measurement Mandate: On the Road to Performance Improvement in Health Care.* Oakbrook Terrace, IL: Joint Commission, 1993.

3. Joint Commission on Accreditation of Healthcare Organizations: *Primer on Indicator Development and Application.* Oakbrook Terrace, IL: Joint Commission, 1990.

4. Nadzam DM et al: Data-driven performance improvement in health care: The Joint Commission's indicator measurement system (IMSystem). *The Joint Commission Journal of Quality Improvement,* pp 492-500, Nov 1993.

5. Quality Management, Sisters of Mercy Health System: *Methodology for SMHS Statistical Patient Outcome Studies* (internal document) St. Louis: Sisters of Mercy, 1991.

6. Bechtel GA et al: A continuous quality improvement approach to medication administration. *Journal of Nursing Care Quality* 7(3): 28-34, 1993.

7. Quality connection storyboard, *Quality Connection* 2(3): 8-9, 1993.

8. Powers SM: How to assemble a patient-centered pharmacy QI program. *Topics in Hospital Pharmacy Management* 13(2): 46-54, 1993.

9. Miller D and Durbin S: Improving patient recovery following total joint replacement. *The Quality Letter,* pp 22-26, Feb 1992.

10. Romfh PC et al: Babies provide focus for quality improvement team. *Clinical Laboratory Management Review*, pp 145-156, Mar/Apr 1993.

11. Goldman DA et al: Hospital-based continuous quality improvement: A realistic appraisal. *Clinical Performance and Quality Health Care* 1(2): pp 69-79, 1993.

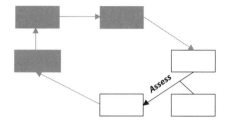

Chapter 4

A S S E S S

Once data are collected as part of measurement, they must be put to use. The first step in that use is assessment. Assessing data means translating data into information we can use to make judgments and draw conclusions about performance: for example, determining current level of performance; identifying and interpreting any variations in process or outcomes that suggest improvement may be necessary; and identifying root causes for the current performance. This assessment forms the basis for actions taken to improve performance.

Figure 4-1, page 84, illustrates how assessment carries us further along the improvement cycle.

This chapter offers concise answers to the essential questions about assessment:

- Why do we assess performance?

Cycle for Improving Performance—Assess

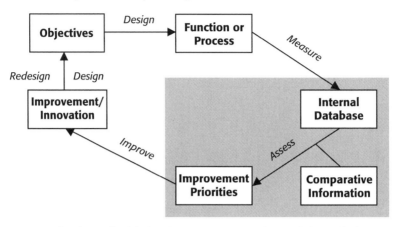

Figure 4-1. *This figure highlights the **assessment** phase of the cycle for improving performance. It includes the comparative information this activity requires and the improvement priorities that result.*

- What performance do we assess?
- How do we assess performance?
- Who assesses performance?

A section of assessment examples reinforces and illustrates this information. See Figure 4-2, page 85, for a summary of important factors involved in assessment.

I. WHY DO WE ASSESS? THE PURPOSE OF ASSESSMENT

Once data are collected, they must be interpreted. This interpretation, or assessment, allows an organization to derive information regarding the level of performance and causes for the current performance—information that can lead to improvement actions.

Assessment is designed to answer these questions:

- Are there problems that need to be solved?
- What processes or functions can we improve?
- What are the priorities among these opportunities for improvement?

For example, when an organization designs a new process, it will measure how that process performs; the resulting data will be compared to design specifications to determine if the process

Cycle for Improving Performance—Assessment Issues

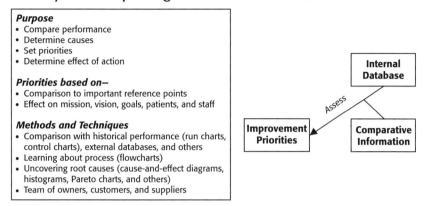

Purpose
- Compare performance
- Determine causes
- Set priorities
- Determine effect of action

Priorities based on—
- Comparison to important reference points
- Effect on mission, vision, goals, patients, and staff

Methods and Techniques
- Comparison with historical performance (run charts, control charts, external databases, and others
- Learning about process (flowcharts)
- Uncovering root causes (cause-and-effect diagrams, histograms, Pareto charts, and others)
- Team of owners, customers, and suppliers

Internal Database

Assess

Improvement Priorities

Comparative Information

Figure 4-2. *These are some key issues involved in assessing health care performance.*

is performing up to expectations and, if not, exactly where it could be improved.

When an organization measures an existing process, it will want to interpret the data to determine whether the process is stable, what the process capabilities are, and/or whether its outcome meets objectives. Assessment of the data acquired can identify the types of variation in the processes and point out potential opportunities for improvement. Even if a process is stable, the data can be assessed to find possible opportunities for improvement in the processes' capability. Because of limited time and other resources, organizations will not be able to take action to address all opportunities for improvement. Therefore, assessment also involves setting priorities for improvement among identified opportunities.

If an organization determines that an intensive improvement effort is warranted, assessment moves beyond noting patterns in current performance. This assessment searches for the root causes behind that performance. These causes will be the target of improvement actions.

When an organization takes action to improve performance, it will measure the results. The data from this measurement must also be assessed in order to determine whether improvement occurred—that is, whether undesirable variation was reduced or eliminated, or whether the capability of the process and, there-fore, the outcomes are improved.

Assessment is not limited to information gathered within the walls of a single organization. To better understand their level of performance, organizations sometimes will want to examine external information (such as reference databases, professional standards, and other sources) against which to compare their per-formance.

II. WHAT DO WE ASSESS?

Ultimately, data from all measurement should be assessed to give meaning to the data. First, we will look at what is assessed with data from ongoing measurement. The frequency with which all data are assessed depends on the process being measured, the organization's priorities, and the types of indicators, among other factors. For example, a hospital might assess any transfu-sion reaction immediately, whereas data pertaining to starting times for surgery might be assessed every quarter. For another example, a long term care facility might review data about pres-sure sores every two months and data about residents' satisfac-tion every six months.

At times, information resulting from this assessment will suggest that more intensive study of the process is warranted. This study could include more detailed measurement and assess-ment, or it could entail more intensive analysis of the data available. More intensive assessment (or measurement and assess-ment) is triggered as follows:

- By important single events (such as those identified by sentinel-event indicators);
- By a performance level that varies undesirably from an absolute level established by the organization (sometimes called a "threshold for evaluation"); and
- By patterns/trends that significantly and undesirably vary from those expected, based on appropriate statistical analysis (for example, an organization may decide to initiate more intensive assessment when performance is two standard deviations below its mean performance).

More intensive assessment (or measurement and assessment) is also triggered

- when the organization's performance significantly and undesirably varies from that of other organizations or from recognized standards; and
- when the organization wishes to improve already acceptable performance levels.

Finally, Joint Commission standards for hospitals identify these outcomes that should trigger in-depth assessment:

- Patterns in, or significant discrepancies between, preoperative and postoperative diagnoses;
- Confirmed transfusion reactions; and
- Significant adverse drug reactions.

III. HOW DO WE ASSESS? TOOLS AND METHODS FOR ASSESSMENT

The primary goals of assessment, as mentioned earlier, are to determine the level of performance and areas where performance can be improved, to provide information that helps set priorities for improvement, to suggest how improvement may take place, and to determine whether actions actually result in such improvement. In general, accomplishing those purposes involves comparing performance with the organization's historical performance, with performance of other organizations, and with "best practices." The following sections show how various tools are used to assess performance.

Assessing Current Performance

When assessing the organization's current performance (and the effectiveness of improvement actions) data from measurement are compared to some reference point. These reference points may include

- historical patterns of performance in the organization;
- the performance of other organizations provided in external reference databases;
- practice guidelines/parameters or policies and procedures; and
- desired performance targets, specifications, or thresholds.

Historical patterns of performance in the organization

When an organization has accumulated a sufficient amount of data, it will be able to compare current performance to historical patterns. This comparison can take many forms. For example, organizations may compare current performance levels with levels during the previous year. (They may also compare performance levels for various days of the week, various shifts, or various parts of the organization.)

Perhaps the most common and useful comparison using historical data involves analyzing the variation in a process. Variation is inherent in every process; performance measured by indicators will never be static. Consider, for example, that an organization is measuring turnaround time for stat laboratory tests. The turnaround time cannot be identical for each test ordered. For another example, consider a managed care organization that is measuring the effect of a smoking cessation program. Obviously, not all participants will show the same result. In other words, results will vary. The goal in this assessment is to determine the type and cause of the variation.

Variation has two general types and causes. One is called common-cause variation. This is the random variation inherent in every process. In the smoking cessation example, each participant has a variety of factors that affect his or her ability to stop smoking: working conditions, family support, smoking history, and so forth. A process that varies only because of common causes is said to be "stable." (A stable process can be improved as well. An example of this follows shortly.)

The other type of variation is called special-cause variation. This type arises from unusual circumstances or events that may be difficult to anticipate. These causes result in marked variation and an "unstable" process. Human error and mechanical malfunction are examples of special causes that result in variation. In our hypothetical program to stop smoking, for instance, a special cause of variation might be a counselor who misses a session or a participant and counselor who do not speak the same language. Special causes of variation must be identified and eliminated; however, removing a special cause will only eliminate

Run Chart

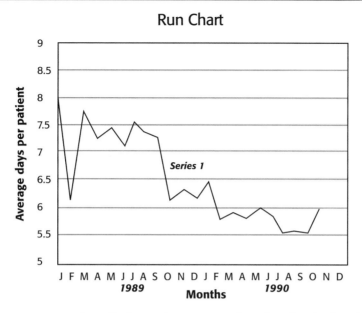

Figure 4-3. *A run chart displays points on a graph to show levels of performance over time.*

aberrant performance, not improve the basic level of performance. A more substantive improvement in performance comes from studying the process and improving its design.

Three tools are especially helpful in comparing performance with historical patterns and assessing variation and stability: *run charts*, *control charts*, and *histograms*.

Run charts. A run chart plots points on a graph to show levels of performance over time. A run chart identifies trends, including movement away from an average. It can show performance needing improvement and can show whether an improvement action has resulted in improvement. Figure 4-3 illustrates a run chart and offers instructions on how to create one. The example in this figure shows the average length of stay per month before and after a process was redesigned.

Control charts. A control chart is a run chart with statistically derived limits of variation added. Thus, a control chart shows variation in a process and indicates whether the variation is due to special or common causes. When performance variation is random and stays within the upper and lower control limits, the causes of

Control Chart

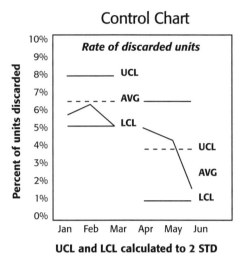

UCL and LCL calculated to 2 STD

Figure 4-4. *A control chart is a run chart with an upper and lower control limit on either side of the average. These limits are determined using certain statistical rules; they are usually two or three standard deviations from the mean. These limits are not the **desired** upper and lower limits (those would be called **specification** limits). They are designed not to say whether the process is running at the desired level, only whether it is statistically in control. This example of a control chart shows the rate of discarded blood units. Notice that as the average performance shifts, so do the control limits. **Source:** Bessley J et al: How we implemented TQM in our laboratory and our blood bank.* Clinical Laboratory Management Review, *May/June 1993, p 222. Copyright Clinical Laboratory Management Association. Used with permission.*

the variation are common causes. When performance jumps outside the upper or lower control limits, or demonstrates specific predictable patterns within the control limits, the variation is due to a special cause. Figure 4-4 gives an example of a control chart.

Histograms. A histogram shows the patterns of variation in a process or its outcomes. For instance, laboratory response times will vary for different circumstances (time of day, number of requests, number of staff, and so forth). This variation may seem unpredictable, but it generally follows some pattern; the range of variation is predictable. In most cases, the variation falls into a normal distribution. For example, perhaps we expect laboratory response between 15 and 30 minutes. At times, however, the distribution is not normal. This may signal the need for further evaluation. Histograms illustrate these ranges of variation. Figure 4-5, page 91 illustrates four types of distribution shown by a histogram.

Types of Variation Shown in Histograms

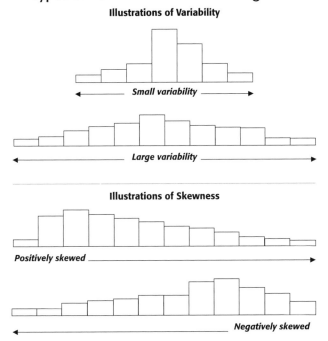

Illustrations of Variability

◄———— *Small variability* ————►

◄———— *Large variability* ————►

Illustrations of Skewness

Positively skewed ————————————————►

◄———————————————— *Negatively skewed*

Figure 4-5. *These histograms show four types of variation distribution: small, large, positively skewed, and negatively skewed. Ideally, the distribution is symmetrical and the variation small.* **Source:** The Memory Jogger™, *p 37. Copyright 1988 GOAL/QPC, 13 Branch Street, Methuen, MA 01844. Tel 508/685-3900. Used with permission.*

External reference databases. In addition to comparing performance within their own boundaries, organizations may compare their performance with that of other organizations. This expanded comparison can help an organization draw conclusions about its own performance and increase opportunities to learn about different methods to design and carry out processes. External reference databases containing aggregate data from many organizations take various forms. One example of an external database is the Joint Commission's IMSystem, described in the previous chapter. The aggregate, risk-adjusted data about specific indicators can help each organization decide how to set priorities for improvement: is its current performance inside or outside the expected range? Health care systems often have systemwide databases that feed information about certain indicators (for example, outcomes and costs of certain treatments) back to member organizations for use in their individual performance improvement activities. Payers also aggregate information about performance and cost, as do states and the federal government.

Practice guidelines/parameters. Practice guidelines/parameters, critical paths, and other scientifically based descriptions of patient care processes are very useful reference points for comparison. Whether these descriptions are developed by professional societies or in-house practitioners, they can represent an expert consensus, based on the evidence in the literature, about the expected practices for a given diagnosis, treatment, or procedure. Assessing variation from these descriptions of clinical processes can help an organization identify opportunities for improvement. (Critical paths are described in more detail in Chapter 5.)

Desired performance targets. Organizations may also establish targets, specifications, or thresholds for evaluation against which they compare current performance. Such levels can be derived from professional literature, expert opinion within the organization, or customer requirements. For example, a medical staff may select a target rate of "vaginal birth after cesarean sections" based on the clinical literature; assessment and improvement would strive to help the organization meet that target.

Determining Root Causes for Current Performance

A more intensive type of assessment requires learning what factors cause or explain the current performance. This knowledge is gained by studying a process; learning its steps and decision points; identifying the various people, actions, and equipment required for the process' outcome; finding links between variables in performance; and ranking the frequency of causes.

A number of tools exist to help this study; these include *flowcharts, cause-and-effect diagrams, scatter diagrams,* and *Pareto charts.*

Flowcharts. A flowchart depicts the sequence of steps performed in a specific process. One use of a flowchart is to identify the actual path that a process follows, as opposed to the one that may be defined in the policies and procedures manual. By docu-

Flowchart

This procedure will help you create a flowchart:

1. Decide on the starting and ending points of the process.

2. Brainstorm to record all the activities and decision points involved in the process. The brainstorming should be done by those people familiar with the various parts of the process.

3. Arrange activities and decision points in sequence.

4. Using this information, create a flowchart. Place each activity in a box and each decision point in a diamond. Connect them with lines and arrows to indicate the flow of the process.

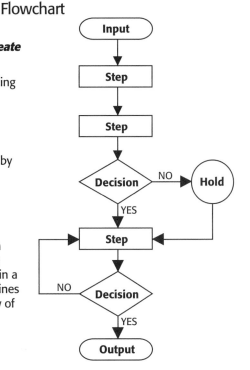

Figure 4-6. *A flowchart illustrates the sequence of steps that a process follows.*

menting the process in a flowchart, a team can identify redundancies, inefficiencies, misunderstandings, waiting loops, and inspection steps; these are the areas that create the headaches and discrepancies in most processes.

Another use of a flowchart is to gain understanding about how the process should be performed. Once the actual process is illustrated in the flowchart, the team can create a flowchart to show the ideal path the process should take.

Teams can use flowcharts at several crucial stages:

- When designing new processes;
- When designing a method for measuring a process;
- When identifying problems;
- When analyzing problems to determine causes; and
- When planning solutions.

See Figure 4-6 for instructions on creating a flowchart along with a generic example.

Cause-and-Effect Diagram

To create a cause-and-effect diagram, follow this procedure:

1. Place the outcome (or problem statement) on the right side of the paper, halfway down; draw a horizontal line across the paper with an arrow pointing to the outcome.

2. Determine general, major categories for the causes; connect them to the horizontal line with diagonal lines.

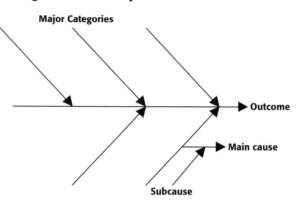

3. Note the major causes and place them under the general categories. The team will need a brainstorming session to determine the major causes.

4. List subcauses and place them under the main causes. To determine subcauses, ask *why* five times.

Figure 4-7. *A cause-and-effect diagram shows a large number of possible causes of a particular outcome.*

Cause-and-effect diagrams. A cause-and-effect diagram is sometimes called a "fishbone" diagram (because of its shape) or an Ishikawa diagram (after its creator, Kaoru Ishikawa). This diagram shows a large number of possible causes of a particular outcome (often a negative outcome, such as a delay, medication error, and so forth). In addition, it can help focus on some specific conditions requiring further attention and might even suggest some appropriate actions. The process of developing a cause-and-effect diagram can also provide ideas for data collection to measure performance. A final virtue of the cause-and-effect diagram is its appearance: it helps people quickly visualize how various components relate to one another. These diagrams are constructed using the experience and expertise of the process' owners, customers, and suppliers.

Figure 4-7 provides step-by-step guidance on building a cause-and-effect diagram, along with a generic illustration.

Scatter Diagram

Follow this procedure to create a scatter diagram:

1. Decide on which two variables will be tested. The team should select two variables it suspects are related.

2. Collect 50 to 100 paired samples of data and record them on the data sheet.

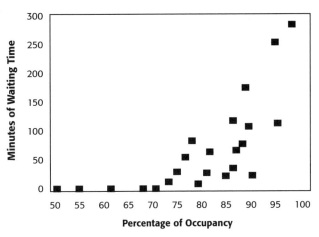

3. Draw the horizontal and vertical axes, noting which variable is represented by each.

4. Plot the variables on the graph.

Figure 4-8. *A scatter diagram illustrates the relationship between two variables.*

Scatter diagrams. Another useful assessment tool is the scatter diagram. This diagram illustrates the relationship between two variables. A scatter diagram may not conclusively prove a relationship, but it can offer some convincing evidence. Groups use scatter diagrams when they want to test a theory about the relationship between two variables, when they analyze raw data, and when they assess an action taken to improve performance. In a scatter diagram, each variable is assigned an axis; points where the variables intersect are marked with dots. If the points cluster in an area running from lower left to upper right, the variables have a positive correlation; if they cluster from upper left to lower right, they have a negative correlation. Figure 4-8 gives more information on how these diagrams are created and includes a sample illustration.

Pareto chart. A Pareto chart is a bar chart that depicts in descending order the frequency of events being studied. This

Pareto Chart

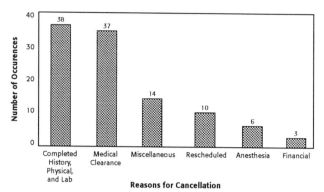

Use this procedure to create a Pareto chart:

1. Decide on the topic of study.

2. Select the type of causes or conditions to be compared. The team must choose the specific factors contributing to the outcome.

3. Determine the standard for comparison—this could be frequency, cost, or amount.

4. Collect data. Check sheets can be helpful for this step.

5. Compare frequency, cost, or amount (as appropriate) between categories.

6. Draw and label the vertical axis with the standard for comparison in increments.

7. Draw and label the horizontal axis with each factor in descending order.

8. Draw the bars to indicate the frequency (or cost or amount) of each factor.

Figure 4-9. *A Pareto chart depicts in descending order (from left to right) the frequency of events being studied.*

useful chart allows a group to categorize occurrences and focus on the most frequent and most important. This chart could, for example, be a natural follow-up to a cause-and-effect diagram. Having listed a number of causes, the group could use a Pareto chart to display their relative frequency. This information would, in turn, help a group decide which cause to address first. See Figure 4-9 for an example along with instructions on how to construct a Pareto chart.

Benchmarking. Another method of assessment is benchmarking. Like using an external reference database, benchmarking involves comparing one organization's performance with performance outside that organization. Benchmarking is predicated on in-depth learning about how other organizations routinely perform key processes to consistently achieve good outcomes.

Although a benchmark can be any point of comparison, most

often it is used to mean a standard of excellence. Benchmarking, therefore, is the process of studying exemplary performance and, to the extent possible, adapting that information for use. When one organization learns of another whose performance is exemplary, the first organization seeks to learn (for instance, through a visit) about the second to study its patterns of care or service for the process in question. The result is often an infusion of new ideas—ideas that never would arise if the assessment remained within one institution's walls.

The organization serving as the benchmark can benefit as well. By discussing the process in question and by re-examining each step and its rationale, that organization may also gain new insights.

Assessing Individual Performance

While most widespread improvement will arise from attention to processes and systems, at times measurement and assessment will identify an individual's performance as the cause of variation. In that case, intensive assessment, final recommendation, and appropriate action and follow-up are required.

Each organization has its procedures for dealing with a problem in an individual's performance. Individual counseling, education, responsibility changes, and required consultation are typical actions.

When that individual is a licensed independent practitioner, the medical staff (including the director of the relevant department or service) is responsible for peer review, recommendations, and any appropriate action. The standards for this process are in the "Medical Staff" chapter of the 1994 *Accreditation Manual for Hospitals* listed under "renewing/revising clinical privileges" and "responsibilities of each department/service director." When the individual is not a licensed independent practitioner, the department/service director is responsible for determining competence.

Although important individual performance issues will continue to arise, it is vital to remember these tenets of performance improvement:

- The vast majority of health care professionals are skilled, knowledgeable, and dedicated; and

- The vast majority of improvement opportunities lie within our processes, not individuals.

Setting Priorities for Improvement

Throughout the improvement cycle, organizations must set priorities for design, measurement, intensive assessment, and improvement. This last instance—setting priorities for improvement—is crucial because of the time and effort involved and the potential effect on organizationwide performance.

Setting priorities for improvement can be seen as a transition between the "assess" and "improve" stages of the cycle—a link between the information gathered in assessment and the initiation of actions to improve performance.

Role of leaders. An organization's leaders play a key role in setting priorities for improvement. They will, of course, need input from the appropriate people and departments/units in the organization, but the leaders are in the best position to view

- the organization's overall goals;
- the availability of resources to address the improvement opportunities; and
- the organizationwide effect of changes in process and outcome.

Changing priorities. The improvement priorities are not static. Leaders will want to regularly revisit the list and update it as necessary. Improvement priorities can be influenced in various ways, including, for example,

- by a sentinel event that requires immediate improvement action;
- by a new or modified strategic direction from the board;
- by patient/family/client feedback; and/or
- by medical staff feedback.

The priorities for improvement should be a living document, responding to an array of changing influences.

Criteria for setting priorities. The following list is a more detailed consideration of some basic criteria that influence improvement priorities.

- The degree to which the opportunity reflects *the organization's mission, priorities, and goals.* If, for example, one of the organization's key strategic goals is to improve emergency services, a project to improve patient flow through the emergency department might be desirable.

- The *resources required* to pursue the improvement opportunity. Some improvements (such as minor procedural changes) require relatively few resources; others require more substantial amounts of time (for example, creating a critical path) and/or funds (for example, establishing a new service). The resources required must be weighed against the resources available and the benefits expected. In some cases, the lack of resources necessary to make an improvement will result in the opportunity being assigned a lower priority.

- Whether the opportunity affects one of the *patient-care and organizational functions* identified in Joint Commission standards. These functions significantly affect the care patients receive and the organization's ability to provide that care.

- Whether the improvement opportunity addresses a *high-volume, high-risk,* or *problem-prone* process.

- The degree to which the opportunity reflects *patients' priorities with respect to their needs and expectations.* One part of performance improvement is to focus on customers—understanding and fulfilling their needs and expectations. In a health care organization, patients/clients/residents are critical customers.

- Whether the opportunity pertains to a *high-impact clinical service.* Such services may include medication use; surgical procedures; blood and blood component use; emergency department triage; hospital, ambulatory, and home care of patients with HIV; care of suicidal patients; use of restraints and seclusion; care of patients on home ventilation support; nutritional support of long term care residents; communication about patient status across service settings; prevention of infection in ambulatory oncology patients.

- Whether the opportunity pertains to utilization management, risk management, and/or quality control concerns. These areas typically are of high priority in health care organizations.

Selection Grid

Priorities for Improvement

Criteria / Issues	Quality of Care	Patient Satisfaction	Staff Morale	Cost	Total
Issue #1	X	X	—		X - 2 0 - 0 __ - 1
Issue #2	0	X	X	—	X - 2 0 - 1 __ - 1
Issue #3	—	X	0	X	X - 2 0 - 0 __ - 1
Issue #4	—	—	X	0	X - 1 0 - 1 __ - 2
Issue #5	0	—		—	X - 0 0 - 1 __ - 2
Issue #6	0	0	—	X	X - 1 0 - 2 __ - 1

Key to scoring
X = strong effect — = weak effect
0 = some effect = no effect

Figure 4-10. *This figure shows a selection grid being used to set priorities for quality improvement. Each issue is examined for four criteria, with scores assigned for each. The answers can help a group see where its priorities actually lie.*

- Whether the opportunity addresses a *high-cost function or process,* or whether the opportunity promises significant *cost savings.* The pressing need to provide care efficiently makes potentially cost-saving changes high-priority opportunities.

  Finally, an organization will want to consider a balance of clinical and nonclinical improvement priorities, with careful consideration of any improvement's potential effect on patients.

  Tools for setting priorities. Two specific tools that may be used to set priorities for improvement are selection grids and multivoting.

  A selection grid can be a useful tool for assisting in decision making based on criteria such as those previously listed. Figure 4-10 shows how this tool works. The horizontal axis of the matrix lists the selection criteria; the vertical axis lists the improvement opportunities. Each person involved in the decision assigns a score to indicate the weight or effect of the particular criterion for the particular opportunity. In the right vertical column, the points are totaled for each opportunity. The higher totals suggest the higher priorities. Responses across the selection criteria may also highlight improvement priorities. For example, if the total was highest for issue #1, but the group did not agree that issue would address the quality of patient care, then that issue may not be chosen as a focus for improvement.

Another tool to decide among improvement opportunities is multivoting—a technique for narrowing a broad list of ideas to those most important. Multivoting is similar to a selection matrix without the explicit selection criteria. A list of possibilities is presented, and each person assessing the possibilities has a limited number of points to assign. These can be assigned in any quantity to any of the possibilities, with the quantity indicating level of importance. Once the votes are tallied, the range of possibilities is usually narrowed to those the group considers most important. This method does not result in a single choice among the possibilities; rather, it allows the best ideas to float to the top.

Other improvement activities. Developing an organization-wide set of improvement priorities does not mean that no other improvement activities take place. For example, perhaps several improvement opportunities related to radiology have been considered and meet many of the criteria, but are not given organization-wide priority. If the radiology department (or other relevant parts of the organization) has the resources, it may initiate its own improvement activities. These activities can use the tools and techniques (such as valid data, flowcharts, customer input) discussed in this book; they may use either a formal or informal improvement process; and they may be carried out by a designated team or by a natural workgroup.

VI. WHO PERFORMS THE ASSESSMENT?

Initial assessment may be performed by those who designed the measurement method or by others with a solid knowledge of

- statistics;
- the process being measured;

- the reference points against which performance is compared; and
- the patterns, variation, levels, and other criteria for triggering intensive assessment.

Intensive assessment ordinarily includes the people involved in the process being addressed: those people responsible for the process, those who carry out the process, and those who are affected by the process. Departmental barriers cannot be allowed to limit participation in improvement efforts. When a process involves more than one department or service, the group improving the process must reflect that cross-departmental activity.

By including the process' participants, an organization not only taps the necessary expertise, it also helps assure the necessary buy-in for the conclusions and recommended changes.

V. EXAMPLES OF ASSESSMENT

The following examples illustrate a range of assessment projects in various health care organizations.

Laboratory turnaround times[1]

Introduction

This example shows a team addressing a specific process to determine whether or not laboratory reports were available when physicians wanted them. The team's assessment includes determining customer expectations and gathering specific data to ascertain whether those expectations are met. The data are displayed to show the degree of variation in the outcome. Comparing performance data to customer expectations or customer requirements is a powerful way to turn data into information.

Example

A team studying turnaround times for routine laboratory reports decides to measure and assess current performance. This is a reasonable starting point because team members, based on experience and anecdotal evidence, do not all agree that delays routinely occur. The team interviews the customers of this process to determine their specifications for turnaround time: by 8 AM

Turnaround Time for Routine Lab Results—Run Chart

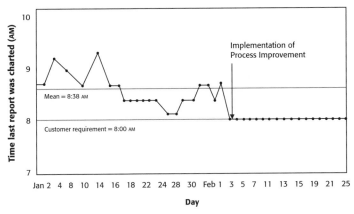

Figure 4-11. *This run chart clearly illustrates the rate of performance before and after changes in the process.* **Source:** *Fisher DE, Gauvin ME: Improving turnaround time for routine clinical laboratory tests.* The Quality Letter, *Feb 1992, p 17. Used with permission.*

the day after the order. The team collects one month's data on turnaround times and plots the results on a run chart. To help the team compare performance to specifications, the chart includes a line indicating the 8 AM target time. The result clearly illustrates the variability in the process' output. Further, customer requirements are not being met. The team continues to use this run chart to assess the effectiveness of the actions taken to improve the process (see Figure 4-11, above).

——— *Treatment of community-acquired pneumonia[2]* ———

Introduction

This example shows that different kinds of assessment occur at different points in the performance improvement cycle. Data collected need to be examined to determine whether anything is "interesting enough" to warrant further investigation. In the following case, variation in mortality rates sparked further study which pointed to a particular DRG. More intensive analysis then pointed to variations in care patterns as a likely explanation, as well as a place for future improvement efforts. The actions to improve care will be tailored to address the root causes identified by this assessment.

Evaluation of Quality of Outcomes

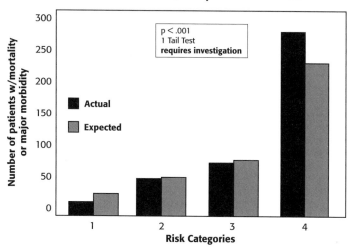

Figure 4-12. *This figure shows the evaluation of the actual and expected quality of patient outcomes in the four morbidity/mortality risk categories.* **Source:** *McGarvey RN, Harper JJ: Pneumonia mortality reduction and quality improvement in a community hospital,* QRB, Apr 1993, p 125.

Example

A three-hospital health system has begun to routinely collect and assess systemwide data regarding major morbidity and mortality. The data are adjusted according to DRG, illness severity, age, and comorbidity; findings are grouped into four risk categories. The data collection and management are performed using a purchased severity rating system, which allows the hospitals to compare their performance with an expected value for each risk category and DRG.

Comparison shows that one hospital's morbidity/mortality rate in the fourth risk category (the highest risk) was significantly higher than the expected rate (see Figure 4-12, above). Further assessment of the data identifies the most likely cause for the variation as outcomes in DRG 89—community-acquired pneumonia.

The data for these patients are assessed further to determine whether variation can be explained by

- the data quality;
- characteristics of the model used to collect and assess the data;
- randomness of findings; or

- patient care factors.

After eliminating the first three potential causes, the assessment focuses on patient care factors. A review of all DRG 89 patients discharged from the hospital within the past year addresses patient factors (for example, age and comorbidities), physician factors (for example, specialties), and patterns of care. This review shows a number of significant variations in medical management and in certain diagnostic, therapeutic, and monitoring activities.

The hospital system believes these findings show a clear opportunity for improving the process and outcomes for a high-risk, high-volume, and high-cost area. Therefore, a multidisciplinary team is formed, which includes

- the system medical director (chair);
- the chairs of family practice and medicine;
- the chiefs of internal medicine, pulmonary medicine, and infectious disease;
- the directors of the emergency, nursing, infection control, and cardiopulmonary department/service;
- the quality improvement coordinator; and
- a medical data analyst.

This team represents the owners of this patient-care process.

The team intensively assesses records of the 35 DRG 89 patients who died and a randomly selected control group of 35 DRG 89 patients who survived; this assessment identifies, among those who died, a low rate of

- sputum culture orders on admission;
- blood cultures obtained on admission;
- prompt antibiotic administration;
- antibiotic coverage for *Legionella* and *Mycoplasma*; and pulmonary and infectious disease consultations.

Each of these practices—according to clinical literature and team members' experience—is important to effective management of pneumonia patients.

Further discussion of these matters uncovers process of care difficulties. For example, primary care physicians suggest that sputum cultures are often not ordered because saliva rather than sputum is usually collected. This observation leads to an examination of the process for obtaining sputum specimens: nurses give patients a sputum cup and ask them to provide a specimen, which the laboratory cultures without first determining that the specimen is indeed sputum and not saliva.

Identifying these key practice issues and underlying causes allows the team to direct its recommendations at these root causes (this example continues in Chapter 5).

―――――――――― *Cost of bypass graft surgery*[3] ――――――――――

Introduction

Assessment or analysis of performance data always involves comparing what has been measured to some reference point. In this instance, the comparison is one hospital's case management practices versus another's. By visiting the reference hospital which had lower CABG costs, the improvement team was able to see first-hand how an alternative approach to patient management works to both eliminate unnecessary care and control costs.

Examples

Two hospitals in a health care system perform coronary artery bypass grafts (CABGs). Their outcomes, risk-adjusted, are of similar high quality; however, the average cost per patient is significantly higher at one of the hospitals. The higher-cost hospital analyzes the data to be sure the discrepancy is not caused by differences in packaging or pricing.

Representatives from cardiac care and quality management create a team of surgeons, cardiologists, anesthesiologists, nurses, and others to discuss the data and study their CABG process. The group develops a flowchart to summarize the current procedures. To study utilization patterns, each member researches specific charge items in his or her area of practice. Although the group believes it better understands its practice and utilization patterns, and although the members identify some variations among practitioners, the group still cannot explain the cost differences with the fellow system member.

The group's leaders contact their colleagues at the second

―――――

hospital to arrange a visit. The second hospital organizes a group comprising counterparts to the first group. During the visit, the counterparts tour the hospital, discussing and observing its CABG procedures. Then the groups reconvene and discuss their findings.

As a result of the visit, the first hospital proposes several process changes, including doing fewer routine arterial blood gases during surgery, discontinuing oxygen therapy sooner, modifying the use of steroids, and reducing the frequency of lab tests such as hematocrits, glucoses, and cardiac enzymes.

Delayed discharges[4]

Introduction

In an initial assessment, discharge data are compared to expectations set forth in hospital policy. Given significant variance from policy, a flowchart of the discharge process is developed to guide abstraction of medical records. Data arrayed in a Pareto chart identify likely interventions to make discharge more timely.

Example

According to policy at this hospital, discharge time is 11 AM; however, ongoing measurement shows that the great majority of patients are not discharged by this time. The hospital forms a team to assess and improve the discharge process. The team includes an admitting clerk, environmental services staff person, hospital volunteer, charge nurse, nurse manager, risk manager, coordinator of management information systems, business office administrative director, vice president of nursing, senior vice president for medical affairs, and senior vice president/chief financial officer.

This team creates several flowcharts to understand and document the discharge process. Figure 4-13, page 108, shows the two key points in this process where delays are noted.

The team next reviews one month's delayed discharges for each nursing unit, noting the specific causes for each delay. Data are tabulated and grouped by cause; the results are displayed in the Pareto chart in Figure 4-14, page 109. This chart clearly shows that three causes are responsible for most (87%) delays:

Patient Discharge — Flowchart

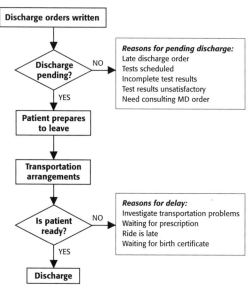

Figure 4-13. *This flowchart illustrates this hospital's patient discharge process. The chart highlights the points at which delays occur.* **Source:** *Bhrany V et al: Improving Patient Discharge Time.* The Quality Letter, *Feb 1992, p 31. Used with permission.*

- Late ride;
- Late discharge order; and
- Ambulance transfer.

The team now can tailor its improvement actions to address these primary causes. The team's improved understanding of the discharge process will help it know exactly what changes will affect these causes.

—————— *Blood culture contamination*[5] ——————

Introduction

In this case study, the initial assessment involves a comparison of the hospital's observed rate to what the scientific literature reports, confirmed by in-house experts. An unacceptably high level of contamination triggers a multidisciplinary team to look for factors that predict high rates of contamination—and they find some!

Example

At this hospital, one indicator measuring laboratory performance is

Causes of Late Discharges — Pareto Chart

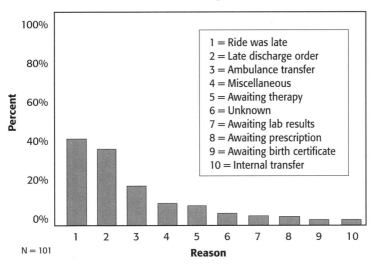

Figure 4-14. *This Pareto chart helps the team see that only three causes are responsible for 87% of discharge delays, thus helping the team focus its improving actions.* **Source:** *Bhrany V, et al: Improving patient discharge time.* The Quality Letter, *Feb 1992, p 31. Used with permission.*

the rate of blood culture contamination. Based on in-house expertise and clinical literature, the hospital has established a target rate of 3% or less for this indicator. Ongoing measurement during the past year has shown contamination rates consistently above that 3% target rate. In addition to this formal measurement, increasing complaints from physicians suggest the need for improvement in the collection process. The hospital selects this process for an intensive improvement project because of the persistent unacceptable performance, the physician dissatisfaction, the costs associated with contamination, its effect on patients, and because traditional problem-solving approaches have not improved performance.

The intensive assessment begins by forming a team composed of phlebotomists, nurses, medical technologists, and physicians. The team first outlines the process of blood culture collection. Next, to identify process factors that may be associated with contamination, the team brainstorms and constructs a cause-and-

Possible Sources of Blood Culture Contamination—
Cause-and-Effect Diagram

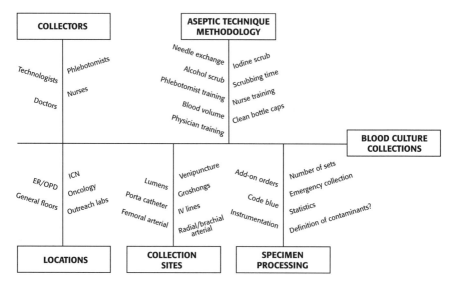

Figure 4-15. *This diagram allows the team to group the various causes and subcauses for blood culture contamination. Based on this diagram, the team collects data to determine the prevalence of various causes.* **Source:** *Lumphrey D: TQM to the rescue.* MLO, *May 1993, p 34. Used with permission.*

effect diagram (Figure 4-15). This diagram groups the various causes under the headings "collectors," "locations," "collection sites," "aseptic technique," and "specimen processing."

The team next collects six months of data to associate blood contamination with the locations, collection sites, and collectors. By far, most incidents of blood contamination occurred in the emergency department, using venous collection, and with phlebotomist collectors. Based on these data, the team can determine where to focus its improvement actions.

VI. SUMMARY POINTS
- *Why do we assess?*
  - To compare performance with various reference points.
  - To determine root causes for current performance.
  - To set improvement priorities.
  - To determine the effect of improvement actions.

- *What do we assess?*
  - Data for all performance measures.
  - Intensive assessment is triggered
    * by important single events;
    * by certain levels and/or patterns/trends;
    * when the organization's performance varies significantly and undesirably from that of other organizations;
    * when the organization's performance varies significantly and undesirably from recognized standards; and
    * when the organization wishes to improve already accept- able performance.
- *How do we assess?*
  - By learning about the process.
  - By comparing performance with important reference points.
  - By uncovering root causes for current performance.
- *Who performs the assessment?*
  - A group that includes the process' owners, customers, and suppliers, with additional expert input (for example, on statistical methods) as needed.

REFERENCES

1. Fisher DE and Gauvin ME: Improving turnaround time for routine clinical laboratory tests. *The Quality Letter*, pp 16-18, Feb 1992.

2. McGarvey RN: Pneumonia mortality reduction and quality im- provement in a community hospital. *QRB*, pp 124-129, Apr 1993.

3. Brewster C, et al: Improving cardiac care: beyond institutional walls. *The Quality Letter*, pp 24-30, Nov 1993.

4. Bhrany V, et al: Improving patient discharge time. *The Quality Letter*, pp 30-32, Feb 1992.

5. Lumphrey D: TQM to the rescue. *MLO Medical Laboratory Observer*, pp 33-38, May 1993.

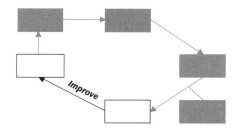

Chapter 5
IMPROVE

This stage in the cycle for improving performance builds on all previous stages. Design, measurement, and assessment lead us to the point where we can take specific actions to improve performance. Improvements that focus on a process can come about through redesign of existing processes or through innovation by designing new processes. Figure 5-1, page 114, illustrates this portion of the cycle for improving performance. Figure 5-2, page 115, shows important factors in this part of the cycle.

I.   WHAT ARE THE GOALS OF IMPROVEMENT?
Although improvement is the culmination of designing, measuring, and assessing, it is not a static goal. Organizations committed to quality do not seek a single level of "optimal" performance, but continuously find and take advantage of improvement oppor-

Cycle for Improving Performance—Improve

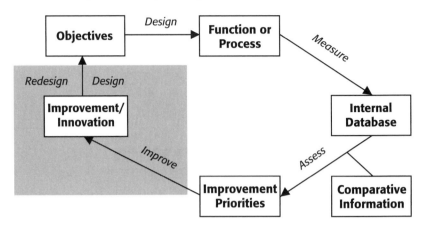

Figure 5-1. *By adding* **improve** *and* **redesign/design**, *one turn through the cycle is complete.*

tunities in all important functions, even ones that have already been through the improvement cycle.

Part of the improvement process is deciding the goals of improvement and the means to determine whether those goals are met. To set goals for improvement, organizations will need to ask and answer the following basic questions.

What dimension(s) of performance will be most affected by the change? To understand the potential effects of the improvement activity, the organization must determine the related dimension of performance (efficacy, appropriateness, availability, timeliness, effectiveness, continuity, safety, efficiency, and respect and caring). At times, an interaction between dimensions must be considered (for example, when a service's availability is increased, the process' efficiency may decline).

How do we expect, want, and need the improved process to perform? The organization (and/or the group carrying out the effort) should set specific expectations for performance resulting from the design or improvement. These expectations can be derived from staff expertise, patient/public expectations, experiences of other organizations, recognized standards, and other sources. Without these expectations, the organization will not

Cycle for Improving Performance—Improvement Issues

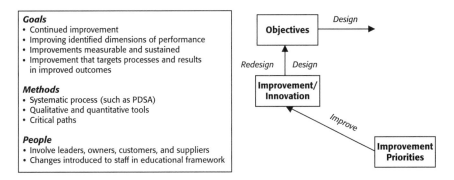

Figure 5-2. *Health care organizations improving their performance address the issues shown here.*

be able to determine the degree of success of the efforts.

How will we measure that the process is actually performing at the level we expect/want? The organization/group will need to measure the performance of the newly designed or improved process in order to determine whether expectations are met. These measures can be taken directly or adapted from other sources, or newly created, as appropriate.

Who is closest to this process and therefore should "own" or be involved in the improvement activity? To a great extent, the success of an improvement effort hinges on involving the right people. These are the people from all disciplines and departments involved in the process being addressed. For example, a medication use project would involve appropriate representatives from the medical staff, nursing, pharmacy, and administration. Organizations will also want to make sure the most appropriate group owns, or is responsible for, the project. Using the medication use example, a project about emergency drug distribution might be under the pharmacy's domain, whereas a project to improve use patterns of certain antibiotics might be owned by the medical staff, or the medical staff in conjunction with the pharmacy. Process issues related to medication administration may be the primary responsibility of nursing.

Processes and Individuals

Improvement actions should be directed primarily at processes. As stated earlier in this book, process improvement holds the greatest opportunity for significant change, whereas changes related to an individual's performance may have limited effect. In health care, as in other endeavors, effective people often find themselves carrying out ineffective processes.

Individual performance cannot, however, be ignored. In health care, the possible consequences of skill, knowledge, or judgment problems are grave. Therefore, when measurement and assessment direct attention to an individual's performance, appropriate action must be taken. Often, that action involves counseling or education, assuming that these professionals can improve and want to improve. In the occasional cases when a health care professional will not or cannot address performance problems, other actions are necessary in accordance with policies and procedures. These actions may include modifying clinical privileges or job assignment.

Hospitals should consult standards in the "Medical Staff," "Leadership," and "Management of Human Resources" chapters of the *Accreditation Manual for Hospitals* for more information on individual performance. (The "Management of Human Resources" chapter will appear in the 1995 edition of the manual.)

II. HOW DO WE IMPROVE PROCESSES? TOOLS AND METHODS FOR IMPROVEMENT AND INNOVATION

Having the goals of improvement firmly defined, and having improvement priorities identified, the organization can begin planning and carrying out improvements and innovations. A standard, yet flexible, process for carrying out these changes should help leaders and others assure that actions address root causes, involve the right people, and result in desired and sustained changes.

The basic aspects of any improvement process are
- planning the change;
- testing the change;
- studying its effects; and
- implementing changes that are determined to be worthwhile.

The Scientific Method

Many readers will readily associate the preceding activities with the scientific method. Indeed, the scientific method is the fundamental, inclusive paradigm for change:

- Determine what we know now (about a process, problem, topic of interest).
- Decide what we want to learn/change/improve.
- Develop a hypothesis about how the change can be accomplished.
- Test the hypothesis.
- Assess the effect of the test; compare results "before versus after" or "traditional versus innovative."
- Implement successful improvements or re-hypothesize and conduct another experiment.

This orderly, logical, inclusive process for improvement will serve organizations well as they attempt to assess and improve performance.

Plan-Do-Study-Act

A well-established process for improvement that is based on the scientific method is the *plan-do-study-act cycle* (also called the plan-do-check-act cycle). This process is ascribed to Walter Shewhart, a quality improvement pioneer with Bell Laboratories in the 1920s and 1930s. The process is also widely associated with W. Edwards Deming, a student and later a colleague of Shewhart. Deming made the plan-do-study-act cycle central to his influential teachings about quality. The cycle is compelling in its logic, simplicity, and continuous nature. A brief explanation of this process should help readers not already familiar with plan-do-study-act to understand and use the cycle. Figure 5-3, page 118, illustrates this cycle.

Plan. In this context, "plan" means to create an operational plan for testing the chosen improvement action. Planning involves determining who will be involved in the test, what they need to know to participate in the test, the testing timetables, how the test will be implemented, why the idea is being tested, what the success factors are, and how the process and outcomes of the test

PDSA Cycle

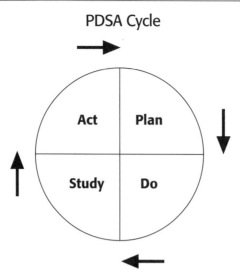

Figure 5-3. *This cycle—also called the Shewhart Cycle—is useful in planning, testing, assessing, and implementing an action to improve a process.* **Source:** *Shewhart, WA:* Economic Control of Quality Manufactured Product *New York: Van Nostrand, 1931.*

will be measured and assessed. The list of proposed improvement actions should be narrowed to a number that can be reasonably tested—perhaps between two and four.

Do. "Do" means to implement the pilot test and collect actual performance data.

Study. "Study" means to analyze the data collected during the pilot test. This analysis seeks to answer this question: Was the improvement action entirely successful, partially successful, or not successful in achieving the desired outcome(s)? To determine the degree of success, compare actual test performance to desired performance targets and to baseline results achieved using the established process.

Act. The next step of the process is to take action. If the pilot test is not successful, the cycle repeats. Once actions have been shown to be successful, they are made part of standard operating procedure. The process does not stop here. The effectiveness of the action continues to be measured and assessed to be sure improvement is maintained.

Tools for Making Improvements

Because improvements are a natural outgrowth of measurement and assessment, the tools used in those activities are as important in taking action to improve processes. For example,

- *brainstorming* can be used to create ideas for improvement actions;
- *multivoting* and *selection grids* can help a group decide among various possible improvement actions;
- *flowcharts* can help a group design a new process or redesign an existing one;
- *cause-and-effect diagrams* can indicate possible causes that an action should address;
- *Pareto charts* can show the effect of improvement actions on root causes;
- *run charts* and *control charts* can measure the effect of a process change; and
- *histograms* can show changes in variation as the result of an action.

Further details and examples of these tools are available in Chapters 3 and 4.

Critical Paths

One significant improvement method not yet discussed is the critical path (also referred to as "clinical paths" and clinical or critical "pathways"). Developing a critical path involves gathering the process' owners, customers, and suppliers to design a new process or to describe, systematize, and standardize a current process. A critical path is an excellent way to devise the process for a new service or completely redesign an existing process that the organization believes needs substantive change. One advantage of a critical path is the opportunity to start fresh, cast aside traditional but not particularly effective procedures, and research and implement the best practices.

Critical paths offer a systematic, flexible guide for patient care that can start before admission and continue after discharge. The guide can be used by physicians, nurses, and other staff to guide—

but not mandate—the patient care process. Critical paths are designed by those involved in the process. Thus, patients, physicians, nurses, technicians, and others assemble to offer their unique perspectives and expertise and to reach consensus on the process.

Selecting the process. The initial step in creating a critical path is choosing a process to standardize. If the hospital is planning to launch a new service, the process may select itself. If, however, the hospital wants to redesign an existing process, the choice of process is far from self-evident. The wide range of diagnoses, conditions treated, and procedures performed by any health care organization is overwhelming. In general, a likely candidate for redesign will be one that is high volume, high risk, problem prone, especially interesting to staff, important to patients, and/or key to the organization's mission. Another factor that must be considered is cost. Although cost should not be the only factor that determines which process to address, the potential savings through improved efficiency is a strong and valid reason for embarking on a critical path project. (The suggestions for setting priorities in Chapter 4, pages 98-101, will also be helpful in choosing processes that will be the subject of a critical path.)

Define the diagnosis, condition, or procedure. An appropriately defined process (and patient population) will simplify critical path development. A process that is too broadly defined will cause confusion as the team attempts to identify the various steps and tasks, and will result in a path that is either too complex or too vague. Conversely, a process that is too narrowly defined can result in a path that applies in only a limited number of cases.[1,2]

Form a team. The group that creates the critical path must represent all disciplines involved in the process. For example, a team developing a critical path related to an orthopedic surgery procedure would include at least representatives of orthopedic surgery, nursing, administration, and physical therapy. At one medical center, a critical path team for total hip replacement began with assigned representatives and grew to include social work, home health, dietary, pharmacy, x-ray, escort, blood bank services, and nonsurgical nursing representatives.[3] The scope of the process will help determine team members.

Another valuable perspective comes from patients, clients, and families. The team should elicit information from the people that the process was designed to benefit. Similarly, if other parties are involved but not team members, their input will also need to be elicited.

Create the critical path. The various team members will need to reach consensus on the key activities involved in each stage of the care process. Members will draw on their experience, their knowledge, existing clinical literature and practice guidelines, and patient perspectives. When varying styles or methods of care arise—as they inevitably will—the team should not panic. The resulting discussion can yield important knowledge about patient care. The group should use consensus-building tools and skills to create a path that all team members support. If varied practice patterns are such that the group cannot reach consensus, the path should not dictate one approach over the other; separate paths can be developed when necessary.[2]

Some organizations draft a path and then let the involved physicians review it, whereas other organizations involve physicians in the team. Of course, physician involvement with the team saves time and makes the physicians a more active part of consensus building.[1]

Reports on the time needed to develop a critical path vary from two hours to four months.[3] Organizations should be prepared for a significant commitment of time.

The path need not be limited to clinical activities. For example, a critical path addressing acute care can include, as appropriate, prehospital and posthospital steps, registration, transport, and all other important related activities. In addition, critical paths can include outcomes.

Despite the complexity of the processes involved, teams should attempt to make their paths as concise as possible—one page is ideal—so they will be practical tools in daily practice. Figure 5-4, page 122, depicts a critical path for dementia patients.

Results. At all stages of the care process, health care professionals can refer to critical paths. These documents should be available in all the relevant work areas and departments and to all

Dementia Critical Path—Excerpt

M = Met
U = Unmet
N = Not applicable

Expected LOS:_____   DRG:_____   Date:_____

Shift/Day/Week	Days 5-8	M	U	N	Days 9-12	M	U	N	D/C Outcomes	M	U	N
Consults	- Psych test complete with verbal report (MD) - OT cognitive testing complete (AT)				- Psych test written report back				- Pt/Family will verbalize understanding of results of consult evaluations (T)			
Measurements/ Treatments					- Assessments for depression, Possible psychosis, substance abuse Medical status, elimination pattern ADLs & Nutritional status complete (T)							
Tests					- Tests to R/O reversible cause complete (MD) - Appropriate lab work complete (MD)							
Activity/ Safety					- Sleep pattern stable (RN)				- Pt/Family will demonstrate knowledge of patient needs regarding mobility, self-care, and safety factors (T)			
Diet/ Hydration					- Nutrition/Hydration stable (RN)				- Pt/Family able to demonstrate knowledge of patient's nutritional needs (T)			
Medication					- Medication education complete - Establish D/C pharmacy needs				- Pt has stabilized on meds (T) - Pt is compliant w/ meds (T)			
Discharge Planning (Education, Psych/Soc, homecare, etc)					- Disposition finalized (SW) - Guardian eval complete (SW) - Support agency referrals complete (HHC, MOW) (T) - Output f/u in place (T) - D/C instructions given (T)				- Pt/Family demonstrates knowledge of f/u plan (T) - Pt/Family demonstrates knowledge of financial coverage (T)			
Special Needs: TX of conc med probs	- Problematic behaviors stable (T)								- Pt/Family demonstrates knowledge of advanced directive (T)			
Variance Facts/ Analysis												
Plan												
Signatures & Initials												

Suicide Attempts:_____   Transfer to/from a med/surg unit_____   Re-admits:_____

Patient Falls:_____   Treatment of concurrent medical problems/diagnoses_____

Figure 5-4. *This figure shows one part of a critical path outlining treatment of dementia patients. The path is organized by treatment days and by care process (for example, tests, diet)* **Source:** *Medical Center Hospital of Vermont. Used with permission.*

involved personnel. Only when the paths are put to daily use as a framework for care can their full effect be felt. Critical paths are also valuable for patients; they can increase patients' knowledge and sense of partnership with providers.[1,2,3]

See pages 147-149 in the following chapter for an example of critical path development and use.

III. WHO TAKES IMPROVEMENT ACTIONS?

As with other parts of the improvement cycle, involving the right people is essential. The process for taking action consists of several parts, each of which has different players.

Designing the Action

In general, the group that has measured and assessed the process is in the best position to design the improvements. This group should include those who carry out the process and those affected by the process and therefore should have the necessary expertise to recommend improvements.

Approving Recommended Actions

The scope of an action and its potential effects will determine who approves the change. When substantial resources and significant effect are involved, the organization's leaders will usually have to approve the action, after assessing its potential benefits and the resources involved. In many cases, a solution will be relatively simple to implement—for example, shifting duties within a department. Such a change usually can be approved by the appropriate supervisor. It is important to remember that if a group has obtained the necessary input and buy-in while devising an improvement, the approval should come readily.

Testing the Action

The action should be tested under "real world" conditions, involving staff who will actually be carrying out the improved process. The group or team that devised the action usually will measure the effects with the same methods used to establish a performance baseline.

Implementing the Action

Full-scale implementation of a process change has the potential to change the activities of many people. Although those changes should be positive, perhaps eagerly anticipated, any change can create anxiety. Therefore, the group responsible for the process change must take care to communicate the changes in an effective, empathic, comprehensive manner. The changes should be presented to all people involved in an educational, nonthreatening way. Cooperation is essential for changes to succeed, but that cooperation will not occur if people believe a change is being forced on them. Care should be taken to prepare people for change and to explain the reason for the change. As with the approval process, an effective team should have already acquired much of the necessary buy-in during the process of measuring the processes, assessing performance, and designing improvements.

IV. EXAMPLES OF IMPROVEMENT

The following examples show several approaches for improving a process. No one approach is comprehensive or is the best approach for a particular organization in a particular situation. These approaches are not intended as the final word on improvement, but as a way to stimulate readers' own ideas for improvement. Each example is drawn from activities in actual health care organizations, condensed, and adapted for this book's use.

——— *Availability of physical therapists for home care*[4] ———

Introduction

This example illustrates that not all improvement efforts need to follow the Plan-Do-Study-Act cycle. Although there is obviously some team planning behind the recommendations, the home care agency feels comfortable enough with the proposals to move ahead with implementation. Note that one recommendation aims at remedying an immediate and pressing concern about meeting patient needs in the short run, whereas the second recommends action to solve a long-term structural problem with physical therapist staffing.

Example

A home care agency notes a significant number of lost physical therapy referrals. Initial assessment of the provision of, and demand for, physical therapy shows both an inadequate number of physical therapists to handle the caseload and delays between the referral and initiation of the physical therapy evaluation.

A team is formed to study the process of fulfilling physical therapy referrals. The team identifies these root causes of the current performance:

- Lack of available physical therapy staff; and
- A nonchalant approach to recruiting physical therapists.

The team's next task is to find ways to address these causes. The team realizes that recruitment must be improved to solve the shortage of physical therapists in the long term. It also understands that a short-term solution is needed to improve the pressing situation.

The team recommends, and later implements, these actions:

- *Long term:* A massive recruitment program for physical therapists in the area. The program includes a scholarship program for physical therapy students in exchange for a one-year to two-year work commitment.
- *Short term:* A restorative nursing program. This program (developed after reviewing state registered nurse and physical therapy licensure laws and other related regulations) provides specifically designed therapeutic interventions coordinated by the physical therapist and implemented by the nurse. The program is designed to enable each client to reach his or her maximum rehabilitation potential. Seven nurses are given intensive education on the program before providing these services.

The restorative nursing program is received well by internal customers—the rehabilitative team manager, staff physical therapists, rehabilitative team secretary, intake nurses, and director. Continued measurement and assessment shows that the agency can manage more physical therapy referrals in a more timely fashion.

Availability of infusion pumps[5]

Introduction

Many processes become needlessly complex as new steps are added. Steps are seldom removed from such processes. This example illustrates that some hypotheses about root causes are not confirmed by actual data and therefore are dropped. A simplified process is tested on a limited scale and when it is found to work well, it is implemented throughout the hospital. To assure that the improvement is maintained, indicator data collection will continue for some time.

Example

In this hospital, the quality council has identified equipment handling as a high-priority function and has assigned a team to select and study one important process within this broad function. The multidisciplinary improvement team decides to address delivery of infusion pumps—a process that has produced frequent delays. To begin assessing performance of this process, the team creates a cause-and-effect diagram that groups causes under four major categories: procedures, policies, materials, and people. The team identifies significant factors in all the categories, suggesting pervasive difficulties in the process. To further understand the current process, the team creates a flowchart. The chart, shown in Figure 5-5, page 127, illustrates only part of the complex process.

The study results in two tentative conclusions: the number of pumps is inadequate, and the delivery process is too complex. The team tests the first hypothesis, but it is not supported: data show that less than one-third of the pumps are in use at peak times. Therefore, the team focuses on improving the process itself.

The team creates a new process (see Figure 5-6, page 128) that simplifies infusion pump delivery. The process requires only one call to request an infusion pump; it locates pumps centrally in the distribution department, and also provides for a certain number of pumps to be kept in inventory on specific hospital units (the number is based on historical data). Responsibility for inventory is given solely to the materials management department. Finally, the team recommends the purchase of ten new pumps (to replace old ones) and the standardization of brands used.

The new process is tested on three floors for three months. The team applies the same measures used to quantify current performance to measure any improvement:

- The time required to receive a pump after it is requested; and
- The number of times infusion pumps are not available.

The pilot test shows a sharp reduction in rates for both per-

Delivering Infusion Pumps—Flowchart

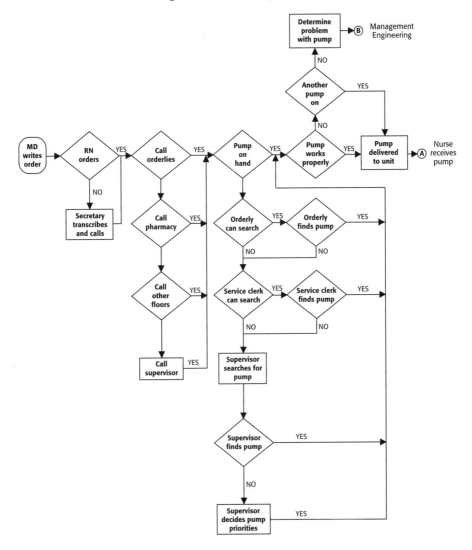

Figure 5-5. *This flowchart documents part of the complex process involved in requesting and delivering an infusion pump. This chart helped convince the team it needs to redesign the process.* **Source:** *Quality Connection storyboard:* Quality Connection *9 (2) Nov 8, 1991. Used with permission.*

formance measures. As a result, the process is made standard operating procedure. Measurement will continue to assess

Delivering Infusion Pumps—Process Redesigned

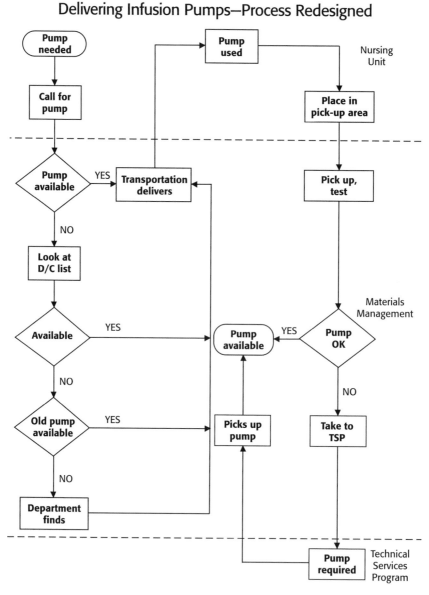

Figure 5-6. *This flowchart documents the simplified, redesigned process for requesting and delivering an infusion pump.* **Source:** *Quality Connection storyboard:* Quality Connection *9 (2) Nov 8, 1991. Used with permission.*

performance. If results are those desired, the hospital plans to apply these techniques to other equipment management processes.

———————— *Community-acquired pneumonia*[6] ————————

Introduction

In the previous chapter, we described one hospital's assessment of the process used to treat pneumonia patients. The team studying the process identified several important aspects that varied from best practices. One aspect was ordering sputum cultures on admission. The assessment showed that physicians ordered relatively few sputum cultures because the process for collecting the specimens often yielded only saliva and the laboratory cultured specimens without assuring they were sputum. Other aspects that needed improvement were blood cultures being obtained on admission, prompt antibiotic administration, antibiotic coverage for *Legionella* and *Mycoplasma*, and pulmonary and infectious disease consultations; each aspect had associated process problems or practice variations. This example reveals how the assessment described in Chapter 4 was used to redesign a patient care process. Since the assessment suggested that problems stemmed from systemic causes rather than people, the team developed a critical path for pneumonia patients and modified specimen collection and laboratory testing protocols. After a test is conducted, further changes are made in one aspect of the medication administration process. Long-term data show the effectiveness of the actions taken.

Example

The team recommends several procedural changes to address problems noted in the current process. Several of the changes pertain to patient management practices and are incorporated into a critical path for treatment of DRG 89 patients:

- Sputum cultures are obtained for all patients.
- Blood cultures are drawn twice from all patients.
- Antibiotics are administered to all patients within four hours; if cultures (blood and sputum) cannot be obtained within four hours, antibiotics are administered.
- Antibiotic coverage of *Legionella* and *Mycoplasma* is strongly suggested.
- Pulmonary and infectious disease consultation is encouraged if the patient has not improved within 48 hours.

The team also recommends the following changes in the procedure for obtaining sputum cultures:

- Respiratory therapists, rather than nurses, collect all specimens.
- Two attempts are made to obtain a specimen (the second with stimulation) within two hours.
- Bronchoscopic collection (as a last resort) can be requested by the attending or consulting physician.
- The laboratory gram stains all specimens to confirm presence of sputum before culturing.

These changes are approved by the medical executive committee with process changes documented in policies and procedures. The changes are introduced to staff through a series of informal educational discussions at medical staff, support service, and nursing department meetings. These discussions are reinforced by seminars for involved physicians, which are conducted by the chiefs of pulmonary medicine and infectious diseases.

During a four-month trial period, data are collected to determine mortality/morbidity rate and length of stay, and whether specific process steps take place, including blood and sputum cultures on admission and prompt antibiotic administration. The findings show lower mortality/morbidity rate, reduced length of stay, and high compliance with all three practice changes.

However, the team re-assesses practices for the lowest compliance area—prompt antibiotic administration—and finds additional opportunities for improvement. When antibiotics are not administered, the team discovers that confusion over the patient's location (in the emergency room or on the floor) and incorrect entry into the pharmacy requisition system are two root causes for this deficiency. The pharmacy staff addresses these problems by stocking the emergency room with the most frequently used antibiotics for pneumonia patients and training those persons responsible for drug ordering, thereby eliminating future confusion or delays.

After 18 months, data show the mortality rate has dropped by 3.4% and average length of stay has decreased 1.3 days. In addition, physicians and other staff involved in this effort are now vocal supporters of the performance improvement process.

V. SUMMARY POINTS

- *What are the goals of improvement?*
    - Continued improvement, not "optimal" performance.
    - Improvements for identified dimensions of performance.
    - Improvements that are measurable and sustained.
    - Improvements that target processes, but address any problems associated with individual practitioners.
- *How do we improve processes?*
    - Use of a systematic method to plan, test, assess, and fully implement the changes.
    - Use of qualitative and quantitative tools including multivoting, selection grids, cause-and-effect diagrams, run charts, flowcharts, and histograms.
    - Use of critical paths to design new processes or redesign existing processes.
- *Who takes improvement actions?*
    - The process' owners, customers, and suppliers devise and test improvements.
    - The leaders approve changes that involve significant resources or effects.
    - All people who carry out the changed process are introduced to the changes in an educational context.

REFERENCES

1. Bower KA: Developing and using critical paths. In *The Physician Leader's Guide*, ed JT Lord. Rockville, MD: Bader & Associates, Inc, 1992, pp 61-66.

2. Zander K: Critical pathways. In *Total Quality Management: The Health Care Pioneers*, eds MM Melum and MK Sinioris. Chicago: American Hospital Publishing, Inc 1992, pp 305-314.

3. Weber DO: Clinical pathways stretch patient care but shrink costly lengths of stay at Anne Arundel Medical Center in Annapolis, Maryland. *Strategies for Healthcare Excellence*, pp 1-11, May 1992.

4. Foreman JT: HealthReach Home Care. In *Quality Improvement in Home Care*. Oakbrook Terrace, IL: Joint Commission on Accreditation of Healthcare Organizations, 1993.

5. Quality Connection storyboard. *Quality Connection* 1(2): 8-9, 1991.

6. McGarvey RN: Pneumonia mortality reduction and quality improvement in a community hospital, *QRB*, pp 124-129, Apr 1993.

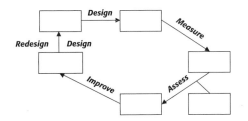

Chapter 6

E X A M P L E S

I. Postoperative extubation of open-heart surgery patients

II. Mammography screening

III. Discharge instruction

IV. Total hip replacement

This chapter presents four examples illustrating the performance improvement cycle. These examples take place in different settings and address different patient care activities. All are adapted from actual experiences in health care organizations, rather than specially created to illustrate this improvement cycle. They give a sense of the range of approaches to performance improvement that are reflected in the cycle described in this book.

The examples also show the wide range of processes that can be improved; the varying complexity of the measurement, assessment, and improvement activities; and the various techniques for improvement. More important, we hope the tenacity, teamwork, creativity, and tangible improvement evident in these examples creates enthusiasm for the possibilities inherent in the Joint Commission's framework for improving performance.

I. Postoperative extubation of open-heart surgery patients[1]

Introduction

This example shows a team tackling a complex clinical practice and improving that process by examining practice patterns outside the organization. The team implements the revised protocol slowly, emphasizing education, encouraging discussion, and allowing flexibility. This example also shows the interplay of measurement and assessment: as assessment provides additional insights, further measurement is often necessary to put the insights into action. Finally, this example illustrates how various types of feedback can inspire an improvement effort.

Example

MEASURE

This hospital has developed critical paths to guide various important processes, including cardiac surgery. The critical path is also used to guide selection of performance measures: length of stay, waiting time, and cancellation rates. Measurement also includes feedback from employees.

ASSESS

Performance is compared to the critical path and variations are periodically assessed. Information from this ongoing measurement shows postoperative length of stay consistently exceeding the goal of eight days. Ongoing measurement has also shown waiting times and cancellation rates for cardiac surgery are high as a result of unavailable surgical intensive care unit (SICU) beds.

Feedback from other sources also identifies postoperative cardiac care as a process needing improvement. Payers desire a lower per-case charge for cardiac surgery. Also, new employees state that in their previous hospitals, cardiac surgery patients are extubated sooner and given lower doses of anesthesia.

These various factors encourage the hospital to form a team to assess the postoperative cardiac care process. The team includes representatives from all areas involved in the process:

- One thoracic surgeon;

- Three critical care attending physicians;
- Two anesthesiologists;
- One pharmacist;
- The respiratory care supervisor;
- Two respiratory therapists;
- The SICU assistant nurse manager;
- Two SICU staff nurses; and
- A quality advisor (from management services).

The team's mission statement follows:

The postoperative cardiac care team will study current practices in our hospital and will study practices in other organizations. The goal is to change the process so we can fulfill our target of extubation within eight hours postop. Decreased intubation time can improve patient care, reduce length of stay, and increase available SICU beds.

The team's first step is to document current practices. The team creates a flowchart to understand the current postoperative process (see Figure 6-1, page 136). The team next collects information on the current process, including

- the average time to wean and extubate patients from mechanical ventilation; and
- the average length of stay in the SICU.

(The team also notes the SICU re-intubation rate, re-admission rate, and mortality rate to establish a baseline against which to compare any changes that result from the team's efforts.)

The team decides to compare its hospital's practices with those at other organizations as recorded in the clinical literature. This study shows that other organizations extubate open-heart patients within 5 to 10 hours after surgery and transfer patients to a step-down unit within 24 hours. The team decides to pursue the cause for this variation.

The team creates a cause-and-effect diagram to find potential causes for prolonged postoperative intubation (see Figure 6-2, page 137). The cause-and-effect diagram indicates the current narcotic doses as a root cause for prolonged intubation and machine-assisted ventilation. The team then collects information on the average narcotic doses currently used, the rationale for

Flowchart of Current Post-Op Process for Cardiac Patients

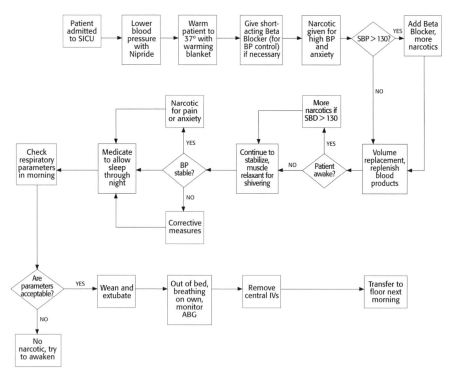

Figure 6-1. *The team uses this flowchart to understand and assess the current process by which cardiac surgery patients receive postoperative care.* **Source:** *Quality Connection storyboard:* Quality Connection *2(3): 8, 1993. Used with the permission of* Quality Connection *and Janice Schriefer, RN, MBA, Medical Center Hospital of Vermont.*

the doses (increase patient stability in the operating room and, postoperatively, increase patient comfort and lower anxiety), and similar practices in other organizations.

IMPROVE/DESIGN

Based on its assessment, the team develops a protocol designed to decrease intubation time. The protocol incorporates a shorter-acting narcotic for use in the operating room and non-narcotic agents to control blood pressure, anxiety, and pain in the SICU. These changes, the team believes, will enable patients to recover more quickly and be discharged earlier from the SICU.

The team is aware of the need to introduce the protocol to

Prolonged Intubation Post-Op—Cause-and-Effect Diagram

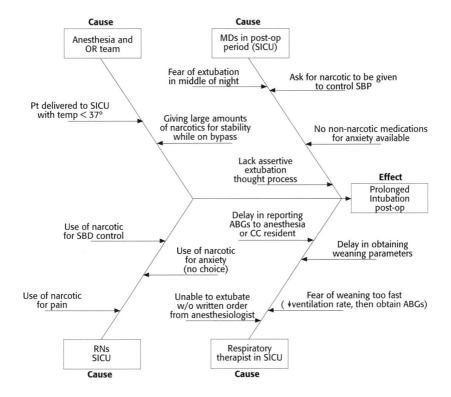

Figure 6-2. *This cause-and-effect diagram helps the team uncover and organize the many factors that can lead to prolonged intubation and a prolonged post-operative stay.* **Source:** *Quality Connection storyboard:* Quality Connection *2(3): 9, 1993. Used with the permission of* Quality Connection *and Janice Schriefer, RN, MBA, Medical Center Hospital of Vermont.*

practitioners in an educational manner. The team designs an educational program for all involved physicians, nurses, and therapists. (The team uses a checklist to assure all the right people participate.)

The program includes

- a videotape showing and explaining the protocol; and
- distribution of the protocol followed by a question-and-answer session.

In any change of practice, some disagreement and resistance

can be expected. The team listens carefully to issues raised and, as a result, makes some comments in the protocol. The hospital decides that practitioners who disagree with the protocol will not be required to use it.

Implementation begins with only the most stable patients. When no complications arise, more patients are included.

The team collects and assesses data on performance related to the new protocol. Each month, the team shares results with staff. The team also surveys staff on their experiences with the protocol. Six months of data show that the average hours of intubation have decreased over 22%, and the average length of stay in the SICU has decreased over 33%. Re-intubation, re-admission, and mortality rates in the SICU have also decreased. The hospital will continue to measure these indicators.

—————— II.   Mammography screening*[2] ——————

Introduction

This example shows the need for several cycles of study, measurement, and assessment. The team probes, tests hypotheses, and probes further in its diligent search for root causes and larger implications of performance. Readers should note that even this extensive description is a condensed version of the team's activities.

Example
DESIGN

As part of its quality management activities, a staff and group model managed care organization has identified a number of important functions for ongoing measurement, including preventive care, ambulatory care, obstetrical care, medication use, and others. Within those functions, the organization measures performance with indicators that address mammography rate, adverse drug reactions, timely follow-up on positive laboratory results, and immunization, among other issues. Based on assessment of the data and consideration of organizational priorities, the quality council organizes specific improvement teams to focus on specific processes. A contract condition for

* The first section—design—of this example is added to the information from the original source.

practitioners is participation in design, measurement, assessment, and improvement activities.

A high priority for the organization is preventive care. The organization recognizes its responsibility—both to patients and to the organization—to encourage healthy behaviors and to intervene early in an illness. Ongoing measurement of mammography rates for women over 40 is part of the preventive care effort.

MEASURE

Measurement has shown the mammography rate at approximately 33% for women over 40 who had visited an internist at least once in a two-year period. The managed care organization routinely compares its mammography rate with that of other health care organizations in the community. Although the 33% rate compares favorably, the organization decides to launch an improvement effort addressing the mammography screening process. Because of the close link between mammography screening and reduced deaths from breast cancer, the organization believes performance rates for this vital process should be even higher.

The organization forms a team consisting of
- an oncologist;
- an internist;
- a nurse practitioner;
- a unit supervisor;
- a health center administrator; and
- the chief of internal medicine.

The team also enlists a pediatrician with experience in quality management to act as a facilitator. The team's mission statement is "to improve mammography screening rates for all women over 40 who visit internal medicine."

Assess

The team creates a flowchart (Figure 6-3, page 140) to understand the current process for scheduling and performing mammograms. The flowchart shows five primary steps in the process:
1. The physician recommends the test;
2. The patient agrees to the test;

Mammography Screening Process Redesigned

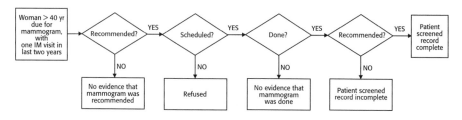

Figure 6-3. *This flowchart documents the process by which mammograms are recommended, ordered, and completed.* **Source:** *Reprinted with permission from Harvard Community Health Plan.*

3. The test is scheduled;

4. The test is performed; and

5. The test report is included in the medical record.

The team refers to data on women who visited internal medicine in the previous two years and compares this data to the steps in the flowchart. According to the data, a few patients drop out at each step; for example, a patient might refuse to schedule a recommended mammogram or a scheduled mammogram might not be performed. The most significant finding, however, is the "dropout" rate at the first step in the process: for approximately 80% of the women who failed to have a mamm-ogram, there is no evidence that the clinician recommended the test. Based on these findings, the team realizes that although it must improve the existing process, it must also make sure the process is actually set in motion.

Next, the team assesses various factors that may be associated with the lack of recommendations for mammograms. The most significant relation is between checkups and mammography: 85% of women in the study group who had checkups also had mammograms, while only 33% of the others had mammograms.

At this point, the team broadens its scope to address the issue of whether these women are receiving other necessary services. The team again refers to data on the study group to determine the services the women receive and consider other variables that may be associated with their receipt of health care.

Significant findings follow:

- The women were not receiving other necessary care and services (for example, almost 90% did not have a Pap smear during the study period);
- Approximately 60% of the women had never had a mamm-ogram from this managed care organization;
- The women's use of medical services was below average;
- The women were not new members; and
- Approximately 90% of the women had a designated primary physician (that is, someone to perform a checkup).

IMPROVE/DESIGN

These findings lead the team to two possible actions to help assure this group receives needed services, including mammography screening:

- Encourage physicians to order mammograms when seeing pa-tients for episodic care (for example, during a visit for back pain or a sore throat); and
- Find a way to make sure the women receive more checkups (which, in turn, will lead to receipt of necessary services such as mammography screening).

After taking the first action, the team sees no change in the mammography rate. The action did not address the root causes of performance and did not create a process that would reliably change performance.

Next, the team designs a process to encourage episodic care patients who have not received a regular checkup to schedule one. Figure 6-4, page 142, illustrates the results described below:

- Before an episodic care appointment, a clinical practice assistant notes the need for a checkup and mammogram.
- When the patient checks in, the clinical practice assistant gives her the appropriate literature.
- In the examination room, the clinical practice assistant reviews the need for a checkup and screening, and answers the patient's questions.
- The patient schedules the appointment before leaving the unit. Before testing this process, the team discusses it with clini-

Process to Encourage Screening—Flowchart

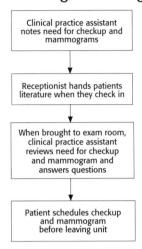

Figure 6-4. *This simple flowchart illustrates the process by which practice assistants encourage patients, during episodic treatment visits, to schedule checkups and mammograms.* **Source:** *Reprinted with permission from Harvard Community Health Plan.*

cians and clinical practice assistants to be sure they agree with the recommended changes. In addition, the team poses three questions that must be answered to determine whether the process works:

- How many patients actually make appointments after receiving the recommendation?
- How do patients feel about receiving these recommendations from clinical practice assistants rather than clinicians?
- How do both clinicians and assistants feel about the process?

Among the first 37 patients to receive the recommendation, only four refused to schedule both a checkup and a mammogram; over 70% scheduled both. The team interviewed patients, clinicians, and assistants to answer qualitative questions:

- Only 1 of the first 11 patients had misgivings about the process;
- The clinical practice assistants, despite the extra work, were enthusiastic about a greater role in the patient care process; and
- The clinicians were pleased to have the extra assistance and to improve the access to care among the organization's patients.

The team recognizes it has not addressed approximately 10% to

25% of women over 40 who are enrolled in the plan but have not visited internal medicine within the two-year period. Subsequent action is designed to reach this group with various reminders.

————————— *III. Discharge instruction[3]* —————————

Introduction

This example shows the wisdom of choosing a modest, yet nagging, difficulty when beginning to use performance improvement techniques. The team involved the customers and suppliers and made sure to get the necessary buy-in before taking improvement actions.

Example
PRIORITY SETTING

In its effort to begin implementing performance improvement principles, this hospital looks for its first process to improve. The hospital is seeking a process that has been prone to difficulties in the past but is not too daunting. The hospital finally chooses to address patient discharge instruction, because

- past quality assurance monitoring has consistently shown inadequate discharge instructions;
- previous efforts to improve performance have been ineffective;
- the process is key to a patient's continuity of care; and
- anecdotal information suggests the process is a constant irritant—to nurses who must fill in instructions not completed by physicians and to patients whose discharge is delayed.

A team from the sixth-floor nursing unit is formed. Members include two registered nurses, one licensed practical nurse, a unit clerk, a social worker, and a pastor. (Physician input will be gathered once the project is underway.)

MEASURE AND ASSESS

To establish a baseline rate of performance, the team reviews a sample of medical/surgical unit charts over a period of two weeks and notes that in 90% of the cases, nurses completed discharge instructions the physicians failed to complete. Average discharge time was 30 minutes.

To understand the causes for this performance, the team

interviews key physicians on the floor about their impression of the discharge instruction process. The results follow:

- 55% believed leaving instructions took too much time;
- 22% did not know about the current instruction sheet; and
- 22% found the current instruction sheet confusing.

IMPROVE

The team implements the Plan-Do-Study-Act cycle to guide its improvement efforts.

PLAN

The team redesigns the current instructional sheet to follow a "check-off" format. This format allows physicians, in most cases, to simply check the applicable element, such as "provide home oxygen." Once the form is developed, the team presents it to the floor's chief physician to be sure he finds it useful and appropriate. Next, the sheet is sent through the hospital's approval process for new forms.

DO

The first step of implementation is to educate all floor nurses and physicians about the new form. Next, the team conducts a two-week pilot test.

STUDY

Results show sharp improvement: discharge instructions are completed by physicians for 100% of the cases, and average discharge time drops from 30 minutes to 10 minutes. All considered, the improvement saves time for nurses and helps clear rooms more rapidly.

ACT

These results are forwarded to the quality council and hospital administration. The sixth floor's results are so impressive that they lead to use of the form throughout the hospital.

———————— *IV. Total hip replacement*[4] ————————

Introduction

The hospital in this example has made a commitment to redesign its key processes. This laudable undertaking is time-consuming, but the rewards are significant. The critical path process shows that improved coordination among individuals—not improved performance by any single individual—can create broad improvement.

Example

This hospital has taken a series of actions to create a quality improvement environment. These actions include training management and staff in the principles of quality improvement, articulating corporate values, establishing collaborative practice and medical staff planning committees, and "de-layering" management to eliminate redundant bureaucratic functions. The effort targeted certain functions for redesign using critical paths. The critical path concept was introduced in management seminars and retreats.

MEASURE

One ongoing measure at this hospital is length of stay for various procedures. This information is especially important because the state regulates the amount insurers may pay for certain procedures.

ASSESS

The state's designated length of stay for total hip replacement is 7 days; however, ongoing measurement shows this hospital's average to be 12 days. The cost and quality implications for this high volume procedure cause the hospital to form a team to improve this process.

IMPROVE

The team implements the Plan-Do-Study-Act cycle to guide its improvement efforts.

PLAN

The team initially includes representatives from the medical staff (including orthopedic surgeons), nursing, administration, and finance. Later, representatives from social work, physical therapy, home health, dietary, pharmacy, and x-ray are added.

The team meets for an hour every other week to determine the ideal process of care for total hip replacement. The team leader emphasizes that the goal is not to revise *existing* procedures, but to create *new* ones.

The team develops objectives, goals, and deadlines to guide its work. Team members are assigned to research and report on the best practices for sub-processes (for example, standard antibiotic prophylactic orders) within their area of expertise.

The team pays special attention to the patient's perspective, ultimately focusing on education and physical therapy during the pre-operative period.

The team designs the critical path one level at a time. The path includes several innovative practices—for example, having both a social worker and a physical therapist visit the patient at home during the month before surgery. The social worker evaluates the home environment in terms of the patient's post-surgery needs whereas the physical therapist evaluates the patient's functional level and helps prepare the patient for rehabilitation.

The path takes four months to develop. Figure 6-5, page 147-149, illustrates a critical path for total hip replacement.

DO AND STUDY

The critical path is tested for one month, and outcomes (including length of stay and functional level) are measured. In addition, the team discusses the process with 10 patients (after discharge) to obtain their reactions. Several patient suggestions are incorporated (for example, reducing duplicated questions pre-admission).

ACT

The communication and coordination fostered by the critical path improve patient outcomes and increase efficiency.[5] Patient outcomes from total hip replacement, measured using the Harris Hip Scale, improved 100% in the two years since the

Critical Path—Total Hip Replacement

	Pre-op Evaluation	Day 1	Day 2	Day 3	Day 4
Consults	PT, SW, Dietary prn	PT, SW	Dietary prn	OT	H & H/home PT
Tests	Visit 1: EKG, CXR, pre-op lab, auto blood Visit 2: auto blood, T & C	H & H (2 hr post-op)	H & H, PT 7A	H & H, PT 7A	H & H, PT 7A
Physical therapy treatment	See home PT eval Visit 2: PT visit —Eval baseline funct —Instruct in exercise, ambulation	Instruct: breathing, quad sets, glute sets, ankle pumps, THR precautions; as tolerates, dangle, stand	Progress exercise: assisted heel slide, assisted hip abd. Instruct: bed mobility, dangle, stand, transfer	Continue progress: bed mobility; transfer; ambulation; exercise (add SAQs) To PT dept, if tolerates	To PT dept: exercise program; ambulation program; transfer training
Nursing activity: (physical immobility)		Side to side, reinforce exercise, dangle as tolerated	OOB hi-chair x 3; observe exercise x 3; bed mobility	OOB chair x 3; observe exercise x 3; bed mobility	OOB chair x 3; ambulate x 2; observe exercise; bed mobility
Nursing treatment		Post-op -> q4hr; NV ck q1hr x 8 -> q4hr; physical assess q8hr; I & O/ pain mgt IV; IS q1hr; teds off q shift; observe drainage; reinforce dressing prn	VS q4hr; NV ck q8hr; physical assess q8hr; I & O; D/C PCA ->oral HL/IS q2hr; D/C hemovac; assess bowel funct	VS q4hr; NV ck q8hr; physical assess q8hr, D/C I & O/ oral pain med; HL/IS q4hr; dressing change; assess bowel funct	VS q8hr; NV ck q8hr; D/C HL; IS q4hr; Fleets enema prn; oral pain med; assess bowel funct
Teaching (knowledge deficit)	Visit 1: orient to unit; view THR video; clinical path; IS/C & DB; pain mgt; equip/treatments	Review IS: positioning do's & don'ts; explain VAS; reason for blood transfusion	Review teds application/ rationale; medication; pathway progress	Review: pathway progress	Review equip avail for home use; pathway progress
Medications (pain)	Consult w/Anesthesia for med taken morning of surgery	Pre-op antibiotics; iron tid; Coumadin hs; MOM 30cc prn hs po; Colace 100mg bid; epidural/PCA	Antibiotics; iron tid; Coumadin hs; MOM 30cc hs prn; Colace 100 mg bid; Mylanta 30cc q4hr prn; oral pain med	D/C antibiotic; iron tid; Coumadin hs; MOM 30cc hs prn; Colace 100mg bid; Dalmane 30mg hs prn; Mylanta 30cc q4hr prn; oral pain med	Iron tid; Coumadin hs; MOM 30cc hs prn; Colace 100mg q4hr prn; Dalmane 30mg hs prn; oral pain med
Nutrition	Visit 1: complete pre-admit nutrition quest; nutrition evaluation	NPO pre-op	50% meal consumed	75% meal consumed	
Discharge planning (impaired home mgt)	Visit 1: SW eval: living situation; relatives; source of income; ability to funct; pt expectations. Home health eval; safety, equip	Identify NH placement/ in-home caregiver prn; LTMA application prn	Level of care if NH needed; ID screen; LTMA application completed prn; in-home caregiver prn	NH inquiries; LOC progress; in-home caregiver prn	Identify equip needs; HH PT ordered; coord meets with family/pt, RN, HHA assigned; obtain pt services
Key patient outcomes	Pt will state: unit/SDA routine; use of VAS 0-10 scale; pt will demonstrate C & DB/IS	Demonstrate use of: IS/C & DB q1hr; abduction pillow and OFT q1hr State: VAS 0-10 less than 5; activity restrictions; rationale for transfusion	Demonstrate use of teds State: meds mgt; review clinical pathway		State: discharge; equip needs

continued on pages 148-149

Figure 6-5. *This critical path for total hip replacement shows the results of an extended effort to design a flexible, innovative procedure for care before, during, and after the procedure.* **Source:** *Anne Arundel Medical Center, Annapolis, MD. Used with permission.*

Critical Path—Total Hip Replacement

Figure 6-5 continued from page 147

Definitions

ADL = activities of daily living

C&DB = cough & deep breathe

CNS = central nervous system

CXR = chest x-ray

D/C = discontinue

DVT = deep vein thrombosis

I&O = intake & output

IS = incentive spirometer

H&H = hemoglobin & hematocrit

HL = heparin lock

NH = nursing home

NV = neurovascular

OFT = overhead frame & trapeze

OOB = out of bed

PCA = patient-controlled anesthesia

SDA = same day admit

T&C = type & cross

teds = anti-embolism stockings

THR = total hip replacement

	Day 5	Day 6	Day 7
Tests	PT 7A	PT 7A	PT 7A
Physical therapy treatment	To PT dept; continue: exercise, ambulation-curb, family instruction	To PT dept; enforce exercise, ambulation, stairs/curb, family instruction	Reinforce exercise, ambulation, stairs/curb, safety; home PT follow-up
Nursing activity: (physical immobility)	OOB to chair x 3; ambulate on floor x 2; observe exercise	OOB to chair x 3; ambulate on floor x 3; observe exercise	OOB to chair x 1; ambulate on floor x 1; discharge
Nursing treatment	Physical assess q24 VS q8hr; teds off q shift; continue pain mgt; NV ck q8hr; assess bowel funct; dressing change	Physical assess q24 VS q8hr; teds off q shift; continue pain mgt; NV ck q8hr; assess bowel funct	Physical assess VS x 1; teds on for discharge; dressing change
Teaching (knowledge deficit)	Teach family application of teds; reinforce positioning do's & don'ts	Reinforce use of antibiotics before procedures; reinforce do's and don'ts	Review discharge instruction
Medications (pain)	Iron tid; Coumadin HS; MOM 30cc HS prn; Colace 100mg bid; Mylanta 30 q4hr prn; Dalmane 30mg HS prn; oral pain med; Fleets enema prn	Iron tid; Coumadin HS; MOM 30cc HS prn; Colace 100mg bid; Mylanta 30 q4hr prn; Dalmane 30mg HS prn; oral pain med; Fleets enema prn	Iron; Colace; oral pain med prn
Nutrition		Nutrional care plan follow-up	Nutritional care plan met
Discharge planning (impaired home mgt)	SW: NH acceptance; coordinates transfer; equip ordered	Discharge plan completed; arrange DC transport; confirm home services; equip checked; confirm home services with family	Patient discharged
Key patient outcomes	Pt state bowel regimen	Pt state discharge plan	Pt state discharge instructions

continued on page 149

critical path is implemented.[5] These improvements result not by increasing the skill of surgeons, but by making improvements in the entire process. In addition, lengths of stay for this procedure have decreased from an average of 12 days to 7 days.

Critical Path—Total Hip Replacement

Figure 6-5 continued from page 148

	Day 8	Day 9	Day 10	Day 11	Day 12-22
Home health: PT activities, teaching		Assess N/V stat, joint ROM, strength, endurance, CNS status, home safety/equip. Teach bed mobility, transfer, gait training, hip precautions, self exercise, energy conservation, ADL education		Assess N/V stat, joint ROM, strength, endurance, CNS status, home safety/equip. teach bed mobility, transfer, gait training, hip precautions, self exercise, energy conservation, ADL education	Transfer to & from car, uneven terrain, stairs without hand rails
RN: activities, teaching	Total assess: family coping; skin integrity op sit & heels; s/s infect, DVT, dislocation of joint, ankle & leg swelling; teach dressing change, univ precautions, antibiotic & pain med sched; observe transfer & ambulation		Assess wound healing, s/s infection, DVT, dressing change technique; teach med action & side effects; s/s to report to MD; use of teds; observe walking with assist device; staple removal prn		Assess wound healing, s/s infection, DVT, remove sutures; draw pro-time if indicated; ambulate with assist device; status report to MD; discharge is indicated
Home health aide: activities		Assist with ADL; transfer bed to chair, chair to commode; ambulate; remove teds; observe heels, back for redness; monitor compliance with abduction pillow		Assist with ADL; transfer from bed to chair, chair to commode; ambulate; remove teds; observe heels, back, etc. for redness; monitor compliance with abduction pillow	Assist pt with shower
PT/SO: activities, outcomes	Family demonstrates dressing change; pt states med schedule, demonstrates transfer techniques & with assist device		Pt/family state s/s of infection; demonstrate ability to take temp & when to notify MD; demonstrate dressing change; rationale for med regimen & side effects		Increased confidence & cadence in gait cycle; independent ADL; free of s/s infection, DVT, joint displacement

CONCLUSIONS

These four examples do not reflect isolated improvement activities. Rather, they show health care organizations

- responding to the challenges of the external health care environment—for example, being accountable for cost and quality and fulfilling community health needs;
- creating an internal environment that fosters continuous improvement—for example, teaching and implementing performance improvement techniques and empowering staff; and

improving processes that are key to the organization's goals in a systematic manner.

No health care organization has fully implemented all the tenets and activities in this framework. However, these brief examples show a laudable pursuit of the goal to continuously improve organizational performance.

REFERENCES

1. Quality Connection storyboard. *Quality Connection* 2(3): 8-9, 1993.

2. Joint Commission on Accreditation of Healthcare Organizations: *Using Quality Improvement Tools in a Health Care Setting.* Oakbrook Terrace, IL: Joint Commission, 1992, pp 78-83.

3. Those minor "nagging little problems" can be very expensive. *QI/TQM*, pp 114-116, Aug 1993.

4. Weber DO: Clinical pathways stretch patient care but shrink costly lengths of stay at Anne Arundel Medical Center in Annapolis, Maryland. *Strategies for Healthcare Excellence*, pp 1-11, May 1992.

5. Bower KA: Developing and using critical paths. In Lord JT (ed): *The Physician Leader's Guide.* Rockville, MD: Bader & Associates, Inc 1992, pp 61-66.

Appendix A

Preamble

This chapter represents a significant evolution in understanding quality improvement in health care organizations. It identifies the connection between organizational performance and judgments about quality. It shifts the primary focus from the performance of individuals to the performance of the organization's systems and processes,* while continuing to recognize the importance of the individual competence of medical staff members and other staff. Last, it provides flexibility to organizations in how they go about their design, measurement, assessment, and improvement activities. Thus, this chapter describes the essential activities common to a wide variety of improvement approaches.

Improving performance has been at the heart of the Joint Commission's Agenda for Change since its inception. This *Accreditation Manual for Hospitals* focuses on the important functions of an organization, and this chapter focuses on a framework for improving those functions. It should now be evident that

- performance is *what* is done and *how well* it is done to provide health care.
- the level of performance in health care is
  - the degree to which *what* is done is *efficacious* and *appropriate* for the individual patient, and
  - the degree to which *how* it is done makes it *available* in a *timely* manner to patients who need it, *effective, continuous*

---

* Throughout the remainder of this chapter, process means a single process and/or a system of integrated processes.

with other care and care providers, *safe, efficient,* and *caring and respectful* of the patient. These characteristics of *what* is done and *how* it is done are called the "dimensions of performance."

- the degree to which an organization does the right things and does them well is influenced strongly by the way it designs and carries out a number of important functions—many of which are described in this *Manual.*
- the effect of an organization's performance of these functions is reflected in patient outcomes and in the cost of its services.
- patients and others judge the quality of health care based on patient health outcomes (and sometimes on their perceptions of what was done and how it was done).
- patients and others may also judge the value of the health care by comparing their judgments of quality with the cost of the health care.

Table 1, page 153 provides definitions for the dimensions of performance. This chapter, indeed this entire *Manual,* is being issued at a time when the health care field is redesigning its performance improvement mechanisms to incorporate concepts and methods developed by other fields. Such concepts and methods include total quality management (TQM), continuous quality improvement (CQI), and systems thinking. The health care field is also incorporating into its performance-improvement mechanisms concepts and methods developed by the health service research community, such as reference databases, clinical practice guidelines/parameters, and functional status and quality-of-life measures. These standards combine many of these useful concepts and methods with the best of current hospital quality assurance activities.

Health care organizations have begun to adopt some of the many approaches to CQI or TQM that have been successful in industry. Most of these approaches give health care organizations' leaders and staffs many powerful methods and tools that are useful additions to those already used in health care. Also, most of these approaches highlight the pivotal role of organizations' leaders and the importance of assessing patients' needs and expectations and listening to their feedback.

Table 1. Dimensions of Performance

I. Doing the Right Thing

The *efficacy* of the procedure or treatment in relation to the patient's condition.
>   The degree to which the care/intervention for the patient has been shown to accomplish the desired/projected outcome(s).

The *appropriateness* of a specific test, procedure, or service to meet the patient's needs.
>   The degree to which the care/intervention provided is relevant to the patient's clinical needs, given the current state of the art.

II. Doing the Right Thing Well

The *availability* of a needed test, procedure, treatment, or service to the patient who needs it.
>   The degree to which appropriate care/intervention is available to meet the patient's needs.

The *effectiveness* with which tests, procedures, treatments, and services are provided.
>   The degree to which the care/intervention is provided in the correct manner, given the current state of the art, in order to achieve the desired/projected outcome for the patient.

The *timeliness* with which a needed test, procedure, treatment, or service is provided to the patient.
>   The degree to which the care/intervention is provided to the patient at the most beneficial or necessary time.

The *safety* to the patient, staff, and customers (and others) involved in the services provided.
>   The degree to which the risk of an intervention and risk in the care environment are reduced for the patient and health care provider.

The *efficiency* with which services are provided.
>   The ratio of the outcomes (results of care) for a patient to the resources used to deliver the care.

The *continuity* of the services provided to the patient with respect to other services, practitioners, and other providers, and over time.
>   The degree to which the care/intervention for the patient is coordinated among practitioners, among organizations, and across time.

The *respect and caring* with which services are provided.
>   The degree to which the patient, or designee, is involved in his or her own care decisions, and to which those providing services do so with sensitivity and respect for his or hers needs, expectations, and individual differences.

Although the standards in this chapter (as well as elsewhere in this *Manual*) do not require that an organization specifically adopt a CQI or TQM program, they selectively incorporate several core concepts of CQI/TQM. Examples of CQI/TQM concepts in the standards include the key role that leaders (individually and collectively) play in enabling the systematic assessment and improvement of performance; the fact that most problems/opportunities for improvement derive from process weaknesses, not individual incompetence; the need for careful coordination of work and collaboration among departments and professional groups; the importance of seeking judgments about quality from patients and others and using such judgments to identify areas for improvement; the importance of carefully setting priorities for improvement; and the need for both systematically improving the performance of important functions and maintaining the stability of these functions.

The standards do not require adoption of any particular management style, subscription to any specified "school" of CQI or TQM, use of specific quality improvement tools (for example, Hoshin planning), or adherence to any specific process for improvement (for example, the Joint Commission's "Ten-Step Model").

The standards in this chapter reflect the need for

- measurement on a continuing basis to understand and maintain the stability of systems and processes (for example, statistical quality control);
- measurement of outcomes to help determine priorities for improving systems and processes; and
- assessment of individual competence and performance (including by peer review), when appropriate.

This chapter has some important links to the other chapters in this *Manual* and, therefore, to other important functions of a health care organization. In particular,

- the chapter presents the performance-improvement framework for use in designing, measuring, assessing, and improving the patient care and organizational functions identified by all the chapters—including this chapter—in this *Manual*. The standards in this chapter point organizations to those functions and processes most directly related to good patient outcomes (PI.3.2 through PI.3.4.2.4) and help organizations set criteria for identifying and prioritizing their improvement efforts.

- the organization's leaders must provide the stimulus, vision, and resources to permit the activities described in this chapter to be successfully implemented. Standards in the "Leadership" chapter identify their role.

- managing the data required to design, measure, assess, and improve patient care and organizational functions requires an organizationwide approach. The standards in the "Management of Information" chapter describe this approach.

- to lead and participate effectively in improvement activities, leaders and staff must acquire the necessary new knowledge. The standards in the "Orientation, Training, and Education of Staff" chapter and the "Medical Staff" chapter set the expectations for education and address this continuing knowledge acquisition process.

Finally, the scoring guidelines for this chapter have been designed expressly to help organizations envision the long-term goals of the standards and make progress toward those goals. The activities described in this chapter will take varying periods of time to implement fully, require varying types and levels of change, and may require resource acquisition or reallocation. Thus, expectations for full compliance with many of these standards will be phased into the survey and scoring process at a pace consistent with the field's readiness.

Plan

If an organization is to initiate and maintain improvement, leadership and planning are essential. This is especially critical for coalescing existing and new improvement activities into a systematic, organizationwide approach. These standards point to the importance of a planned approach to improvement and to the need to have all units (for example, departments/services) and all disciplines (for example, professional groups) collaborating to carry out that approach.

PI.1

The organization has a planned, systematic, organization-wide approach to designing, measuring, assessing, and improving its performance.

PI.1.1 The activities described in this chapter are carried out collaboratively and include the appropriate department(s)/service(s) and discipline(s) involved.

DESIGN

New processes can be designed well if at least the four essential information sources listed in PI.2.1 through PI.2.1.4 are considered. Each of these sources can identify design specifications/expectations against which success can be measured.

PI.2

New processes are designed well.

PI.2.1 The design is based on

    PI.2.1.1 the organization's mission, vision, and plans;

    PI.2.1.2 the needs and expectations of patients, staff, and others;

    PI.2.1.3 up-to-date sources of information about designing processes (such as practice guidelines/parameters); and

    PI.2.1.4 the performance of the processes and their outcomes in organizations (such as information from reference databases).

MEASURE

Measurement (that is, the collection of data) is the basis for determining the level of performance of existing processes and the outcomes resulting from these processes. To provide useful data, measurement must be systematic, relate to relevant dimensions of performance, and be of appropriate breadth and frequency.

The standards in this section address issues such as the purposes of measurement; the selection criteria for functions, processes, and outcomes to be measured; the important sources of data; and the continued role of measuring.

PI.3
The organization has a systematic process in place to collect data needed to
- **design and assess new processes;**
- **assess the dimensions of performance relevant to functions, processes, and outcomes;**
- **measure the level of performance and stability of important existing processes;**
- **identify areas for possible improvement of existing processes; and**
- **determine whether changes improved the processes.**

PI.3.1 The collected data include measures of both processes and outcomes.

PI.3.2 Data are collected both for the priority issues chosen for improvement and as part of continuing measurement.

PI.3.3 The organization collects data about

PI.3.3.1 the needs and expectations of patients and others and the degree to which these needs and expectations have been met; and

PI.3.3.1.1 These data relate to the relevant dimensions of performance.

PI.3.3.2 its staff's views regarding current performance and opportunities for improvement.

PI.3.4 The organization measures the performance of processes in all the patient care and organizational functions identified in this *Manual.*

PI.3.4.1 Processes that are measured on a continuing basis include those that

PI.3.4.1.1 affect a large percentage of patients; and/or

PI.3.4.1.2 place patients at serious risk if not performed well, or performed when not indicated, or not performed when indicated; and/or

PI.3.4.1.3 have been or are likely to be problem prone.

PI.3.4.2 Processes measured encompass at least

PI.3.4.2.1 those related to the use of surgical and other invasive procedures, including (1) selecting appropriate procedures, (2) preparing the patient for the procedure, (3) performing the procedure and monitoring the patient, and (4) providing postprocedure care;

PI.3.4.2.2 those related to the use of medications, including (1) prescribing/ordering, (2) preparation and dispensing, (3) administration, and (4) monitoring the medications' effects on patients;

PI.3.4.2.3 those related to the use of blood and blood components, including (1) ordering, (2) distributing, handling, and dispensing, (3) administration, and (4) monitoring the blood and blood components' effects on patients; and

PI.3.4.2.4 those related to determining the appropriateness of admissions and continued hospitalization (that is, utilization review activities).

PI.3.5 The organization collects data about

    PI.3.5.1 autopsy results,

    PI.3.5.2 risk management activities, and

    PI.3.5.3 quality control activities in at least the following areas:

        PI.3.5.3.1 Clinical laboratory services,

        PI.3.5.3.2 Diagnostic radiology services,

        PI.3.5.3.3 Dietetic services,

        PI.3.5.3.4 Nuclear medicine services, and

        PI.3.5.3.5 Radiation oncology services.

ASSESS

Interpretation of the collected data provides information about the organization's level of performance along many dimensions and over time. Assessment questions include, for example,
- What is the degree of conformance to process and outcome objectives?
- How stable is a process, or how consistent is an outcome?
- Where might a stable process be improved?
- Was the undesirable variation in a process or outcome reduced or eliminated?

In addition to assessing performance over time, further information is gained from comparing data among organizations when relevant reference databases exist.

The standards in this section address the elements of a systematic assessment process and emphasize the importance of asking the right assessment questions and using the right processes and mechanisms to answer these questions.

PI.4

The organization has a systematic process to assess collected data in order to determine

- *whether design specifications for new processes were met;*
- *the level of performance and stability of important existing processes;*
- *priorities for possible improvement of existing processes;*
- *actions to improve the performance of processes; and*
- *whether changes in the processes resulted in improvement.*

PI.4.1 The assessment process includes

PI.4.1.1 using statistical quality control techniques, as appropriate.

PI.4.1.2 comparing data about

PI.4.1.2.1 the organization's processes and outcomes over time;

PI.4.1.2.2 the organization's processes with information from up-to-date sources about the design and performance of processes (such as practice guidelines/parameters); and

PI.4.1.2.3 the organization's performance of processes and their outcomes to that of other organizations, including using reference databases.

PI.4.1.3 intensive assessment when undesirable variation in performance may have occurred or is occurring. Such intensive assessments are initiated

PI.4.1.3.1 by important single events and by absolute levels and/or patterns/trends that significantly and undesirably vary from those expected, based on appropriate statistical analysis;

PI.4.1.3.2 when the organization's performance significantly and undesirably varies from that of other organizations;

PI.4.1.3.3 when the organization's performance significantly and undesirably varies from recognized standards;

PI.4.1.3.4 when the organization wishes to improve already good performance;

PI.4.1.3.5 in response to all major discrepancies, or patterns of discrepancies, between preoperative and post-operative (including pathologic) diagnoses, including those identified during the pathologic review of specimens removed during surgical or invasive procedures;

PI.4.1.3.6 by all confirmed transfusion reactions; and

PI.4.1.3.7 by all significant adverse drug reactions.

PI.4.2 When the findings of the assessment process are relevant to an individual's performance,

PI.4.2.1 the medical staff is responsible for determining their use in peer review and/or the periodic evaluations of a licensed independent practitioner's competence, in accordance with the standards on renewing/revising clinical privileges delineated in the "Medical Staff" chapter; and/or

PI.4.2.2 the department/service director is responsible for determining the competence of individuals who are not licensed independent practitioners, in accordance with LD.2.1.2.5.

IMPROVE

The activities described in PI.3 and PI.4 identify a variety of opportunities for improvement. These include improving already well-performing processes, designing new processes, and/or reducing variation or eliminating undesirable variation in processes or outcomes.

The standards in this section address the elements of a systematic approach to improvement: planning the change, testing it, studying its effect, and implementing changes that are worthwhile improvements.

PI.5
The organization systematically improves its performance by improving existing processes.

PI.5.1 Existing processes are improved when an organization decides to act on an opportunity for improvement or when the measurement of an existing process identifies that an undesirable change in performance may have occurred or is occurring.

PI.5.1.1 These decisions consider

PI.5.1.1.1 opportunities to improve processes within the important functions described in this *Manual*;

PI.5.1.1.2 the factors listed in PI.3.3 through PI.3.5.3.5;

PI.5.1.1.3 the resources required to make the improvement; and

PI.5.1.1.4 the organization's mission and priorities.

PI.5.2 The design or improvement activities

PI.5.2.1 specifically consider the expected impact of the

design or improvement on the relevant dimensions of performance;

PI.5.2.2 set performance expectations for the design or improvement of the processes;

PI.5.2.3 include adopting, adapting, or creating measures of the performance; and

PI.5.2.4 involve those individuals, professions, and departments/services closest to the design or improvement activity.

PI.5.3 When action is taken to improve a process,

PI.5.3.1 the action may be tested on a trial basis;

PI.5.3.1.1 When the initial action is not effective, a new action is planned and tested.

PI.5.3.2 the action's effect is assessed; and

PI.5.3.3 successful actions are implemented.

PI.5.4 Action is directed primarily at improving processes.

PI.5.4.1 Pursuant to PI.4.2, when improvement activities lead to a determination that an individual has performance problems that he/she is unable or unwilling to improve, his/her clinical privileges or job assignment is modified (in accordance with the standards in this *Manual* on renewing/ revising clinical privileges in the "Medical Staff" chapter and on determining competence in GB.1.14 in 1994 and in the "Management of Human Resources" chapter in 1995), as indicated, or some other appropriate action is taken.

Appendix B

The scoring guidelines for this chapter have been designed to help organizations envision the long-term goals of the standards and make progress toward those goals. The activities described in this chapter will take varying periods of time to implement fully, require varying types and levels of change, and may require resource acquisition or reallocation. Thus, expectations for full compliance with many of these standards will be phased into the survey and scoring process at a pace consistent with the field's readiness. (For specific information, refer to the complete scoring guidelines for this chapter in the *Accreditation Manual for Hospitals*, Vol II.)

Goal of This Function. The organization designs processes well and systematically measures, assesses, and improves its performance to improve patient health outcomes.

Scope of This Function. This chapter presents a framework for designing and improving all the important functions identified in this *Manual.*

Cycle for Improving Performance

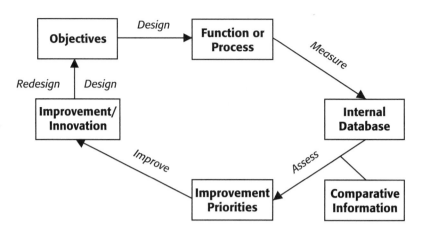

This flowchart illustrates the process for improving performance and outcomes in a health care organization or, indeed, in any organization. The components of the performance-improvement cycle are connected by the actions of organizational leaders, managers, physicians and other clinicians, trustees, and support staff who design, measure, assess, and improve their work processes.* Each of these actions corresponds to the specific activities described by the standards in this chapter.

The performance improvement cycle depicted in this flowchart has no beginning and no end. An organization may start its improvement effort at any point: by designing a new service, by flowcharting an existing clinical process, by measuring patient outcomes, by comparing its performance to that of other organizations, by selecting specific areas for priority attention, or even by experimenting with new ways of carrying out current functions.

This approach is valuable because it is anchored in the real work of health care professionals and in the real improvements that can be achieved to benefit patients and others. This "Cycle for Improving Performance" is not new—it is the scientific method applied to making health care processes and outcomes better. There are many improvement methodologies, such as the Joint Commission's ten-step process, FOCUS-PDCA, FADE, and so on, which an organization may use to structure its improvement efforts.

Finally, this cycle describes only part of the work of an organization committed to excellence. Other critical functions are described elsewhere in the accreditation standards in this Manual. Some functions most closely related to performance improvement include management of information, leadership, and management of human resources.

---

*Process means everyday work—the jobs that you and your colleagues do and are responsible for improving.

DEFINITIONS

assess To transform data into information by analyzing the data.

criteria Expected level(s) of achievement, or specifications against which performance can be assessed.

improve To take actions that result in the desired measurable change in the identified performance dimension.

indicator A tool used to measure, over time, the performance of functions, processes, and outcomes of an organization.

measure To collect quantifiable data about a dimension of performance of a function or process.

measurement The systematic process of data collection, repeated over time or at a single point in time.

organizationwide Throughout the organization and across multiple structural and staffing components, as appropriate.

outcome The result of the performance (or nonperformance) of a function or process(es).

performance measure A measure, such as a standard or indicator, used to assess the performance of a function or process of any organization.

plan To formulate/describe the approach to achieving the goals related to improving the performance of the organization.

process A goal-directed, interrelated series of actions, events, mechanisms, or steps.

reference database An organized collection of similar data from many organizations that can be used to compare an organization's performance to that of others.

relevant Having a clearly decisive bearing on an issue.

sentinel event An occurrence that, when noted, requires intensive assessment.

systematic Pursuing a defined objective(s) in a planned, step-by-step manner.

variance A measure of the differences in a set of observations.

variation The differences in results obtained in measuring the same phenomenon more than once. The sources of variation in a process over time can be grouped into two major classes: common causes and special causes.

EXPLANATORY NOTES

Examples of Implementation, when provided, are meant to give insight into the strategies, activities, and/or processes that an organization may use to meet the intent of the standard(s). The examples are not intended to represent all the implementation strategies that have the potential to meet the intent.

Examples of Evidence of Performance, when provided, are meant to give insight into the forms and sources of evidence that a surveyor may examine or that an organization may present to a surveyor. The examples are not intended to represent all possible forms and sources. Depending on the implementation choices, other sources of performance information may be appropriate. It is therefore important for an organization to consider what evidence will most accurately and clearly indicate its level of performance in meeting the intent of the standard(s).

Plan

For an organization to improve its performance in a systematic, coordinated, and continuous manner, its leaders must describe the organization's approach to improving performance and see that the necessary processes and mechanisms are established. Frequently, the approach, processes, and mechanisms are described in a written plan or as a component of the organization's other planning documents. Performance improvement activities are thus organizationwide and systematic.

A second factor facilitating an organizationwide approach is involving multiple departments and disciplines in establishing the plans, processes, and mechanisms that comprise the organization's performance improvement activities. Patient care is a coordinated and collaborative effort; the approach to improving performance of an important function or process should be also.

PI.1 The organization has a planned, systematic, organizationwide approach to designing, measuring, assessing, and improving its performance.

PI.1.1 The activities described in this chapter are carried out collaboratively and include the appropriate department(s)/service(s) and discipline(s) involved.

INTENT OF PI.1 AND PI.1.1

The activities and processes described in this chapter require a planned, systematic, organizationwide approach to improvement, in which all the organization's appropriate individuals, departments, and professions work collaboratively.

Frequently, improvement activities stay within the structures (for example, departments) and professional boundaries (for example, nursing) of an organization. Although these units/subgroups can be considered "involved," it is clearly not in a "collaborative" manner. Until improvement activities become collaborative (across departments, interdisciplinary), they will be difficult for an organization to plan for and provide for a systematic and organizationwide approach.

EXAMPLE OF IMPLEMENTATION

An organization's leaders decide to incorporate quality planning into their strategic planning process. This will help disseminate the plan and confirm that improving performance must be a systematic, organizationwide activity if the strategic plans are to be realized. Because the plan's goals cut across almost every department and discipline, the activities related to performance improvement will be collaborative efforts.

EXAMPLES OF EVIDENCE OF PERFORMANCE

- Discussions with leaders and staff
- Planning documents
- Meeting minutes
- Training materials

Design

Organizations are often presented with a need or an opportunity to establish new services, extend product lines, occupy a new facility, or significantly change existing functions or processes. It is thus always a goal to design effective processes, for whatever purposes they support; and some fundamental concepts of CQI/TQM can help design those processes well. These concepts lead to four questions:

- Is the process/function/service consistent with the organization's mission, vision, and other plans?
- Has the organization listened to its customers' and staff's ideas about a well-designed process/function/service?
- What do the experts, as well as scientific, professional, and other sources of up-to-date information, tell the organization about the design?
- What databases are available and appropriate to provide information on the performance of such processes/functions/services?

The answers to these questions provide a basic set of performance expectations that can be measured, assessed, and improved over time.

These four questions are also relevant to the incremental improvement/redesign of processes, the focus of the rest of this chapter. The difference, however, is that a "design" approach starts fresh and does not use existing performance data, when available, to overshadow the information from these questions.

PI.2   *New processes are designed well.*

PI.2.1 *The design is based on*

PI.2.1.1 the organization's mission, vision, and plans;

PI.2.1.2 the needs and expectations of patients, staff, and others;

PI.2.1.3 up-to-date sources of information about designing processes (such as practice guidelines/parameters); and

PI.2.1.4 the performance of the processes and their outcomes in organizations (such as information from reference databases).

INTENT OF PI.2 THROUGH PI.2.1.4

When new processes need to be established, they are designed well and consider the basic design information sources described in PI.2.1.1 through PI.2.1.4.

EXAMPLE OF IMPLEMENTATION

In its mission, an organization pledges to provide pediatric care to the community. An assessment of staff and patients demonstrates that the organization's current pediatric services need to be expanded to include pediatric rehabilitation. Staff, patients, and others, such as families and physicians, are asked what specifications should be built/designed into such a unit. Also, any relevant practice guidelines or standards from professional and child care organizations are reviewed. A team is sent to examine the pediatric units in two nationally recognized leaders in rehabilitation care, and a search of reference databases reveals performance measures of how similar units in a 25-hospital system are performing in several key areas. From all these data and this information, a design team establishes how such a unit would look, function, and produce the outcomes of care it believes possible and necessary.

EXAMPLES OF EVIDENCE OF PERFORMANCE
- Planning/design documents
- Design specifications
- Performance criteria for new processes

- Committee notes/minutes
- Discussions with leaders and staff

Measure

Performance measurement is at the heart of all performance improvement activities. Once the existing level of performance is known, the organization can make informed judgments about the stability of existing processes, identify opportunities for incremental improvements in processes, identify the need to redesign processes, and decide if improvements or redesign of processes met objectives.

Measurement, the collection of data, focuses simultaneously on multiple subjects, including

- both processes and outcomes;
- comprehensive performance measures (indicators);
- high risk/high volume/problem-prone processes, including surgical and other invasive procedures, the use of medications, and the use of blood and blood components; and
- other sensors of performance, such as
  - needs, expectations, and feedback of patients and others,
  - results of ongoing activities designed to control infections,
  - safety of the care environment, and
  - utilization review and risk management findings.

The scope of the measurement activities encompasses all the important functions described in this *Manual* and will, over time, measure the dimensions of performance relevant to the function. The interdependence of the important functions, as well as the interdependence of the dimensions of performance, are important in choosing measures. The frequency of measurement is related to the process or outcomes measured and the purpose of the measurement; thus, measurement can occur at one point in time or be repeated over time.

PI.3 The organization has a systematic process in place to collect data needed to
- **design and assess new processes;**
- **assess the dimensions of performance relevant to**

functions, processes, and outcomes;
- *measure the level of performance and stability of important existing processes;*
- *identify areas for possible improvement of existing processes; and*
- *determine whether changes improved the processes.*

INTENT OF PI.3

The questions to be answered by the data are framed before data collection begins to assure that only relevant, useful, and necessary data are collected. A comprehensive improvement program asks many questions simultaneously about many functions and processes; thus, the data collection process is uniform and systematic.

EXAMPLE OF IMPLEMENTATION

A hospital selects to improve the assessment of patients function. In particular, staff wish to know the timeliness of the consultation process and the appropriateness of lab tests. They want to measure the stability of these processes along these two dimensions of performance and gain insight into possible improvements and/or decide if processes should be redesigned. The organization needs to have a systematic process to support completely this priority improvement effort.

EXAMPLES OF EVIDENCE OF PERFORMANCE
- Discussions with leaders, improvement teams, and information services staff
- Review of improvement activities, including questions asked and data obtained

PI.3.1 The collected data include measures of both processes and outcomes.

INTENT OF PI.3.1

A "balanced" approach to measurement and assessment includes measures of both outcomes and processes—outcomes to understand the results, processes to understand what has been done to cause those results. For example, the outcomes of many clinical processes are not evident or measurable at discharge, or they vary considerably due to patient variables. It is prudent to measure the processes that most profoundly influence the anticipated outcome as surrogate measures of the outcomes.

The indicators recommended by the Joint Commission represent measures of both processes and outcomes. These indicators, if relevant, are reviewed and considered for use in developing the organization's measurement processes.*

EXAMPLE OF IMPLEMENTATION

The orthopedic surgery unit in a 1,200-bed academic teaching hospital performs a high number of total hip replacements. The surgeons work closely with the physical rehabilitation program to achieve an optimal level of functioning and ambulation for their patients by discharge. The perception of some surgeons is that their patients take longer to reach that level of rehabilitation. The departments of orthopedic surgery and physical rehabilitation form a team to assess the perception of the group of surgeons. After an initial review, they conclude that the functional assessment instrument used to evaluate outcomes is imprecise and that the process for initiating rehabilitation after surgery is different for those surgeons who routinely schedule the surgery later in the week, especially on Friday. The team decides to initiate more intensive assessment by selecting an indicator that measures the process of initiating rehabilitation. They also decide to select a more precise and tested outcome/functional assessment instrument. The team reviews the indicators recommended by the Joint Commission to see if any address the process and outcome they are reviewing.

EXAMPLES OF EVIDENCE OF PERFORMANCE

- Discussions with improvement teams
- Plans for data collection
- Review of measurement strategies/plans

---

* See Appendix C of this Manual for a current listing of the recommended indicators that have been tested in the development of the Joint Commission's indicator monitoring system.

***PI.3.2 Data are collected both for the priority issues chosen
for improvement and as part of continuing measurement.***

INTENT OF PI.3.2
Repeated measurement over time enables the organization to
judge a particular process's stability or a particular outcome's
predictability. Once a decision has been made to improve a process, measurement becomes more detailed and frequent.

EXAMPLE OF IMPLEMENTATION
The pharmacy department has been measuring the timeliness of
medication deliveries to each hospital wing's floors. It samples a
different floor each day on a rotating basis and has control charts
to display the variation in timeliness. A priority strategy for improvement was developed. During the test period and after the
strategy's full implementation, measurement of each floor in each
wing is done through daily (rather than periodic) data collection
until it is clear that the new approach is effective and stable.

EXAMPLES OF EVIDENCE OF PERFORMANCE
- Discussion with improvement teams
- Plans for data collection
- Review of measurement strategies/plans, data displays, and
  measurement and improvement reports

PI.3.3 The organization collects data about

***PI.3.3.1 the needs and expectations of patients and others
and the degree to which these needs and expectations have
been met; and***

***PI.3.3.1.1 These data relate to the relevant dimensions of
performance.***

***PI.3.3.2 its staff's views regarding current performance and
opportunities for improvement.***

INTENT OF PI.3.3 THROUGH PI.3.3.2

In assessing performance (how well processes are designed or how well they operate), the perspectives of patients, staff, and others are essential. The patients' perspectives are critical, but improving processes and outcomes can also be informed by understanding the perspective of patients' families and/or significant others, surrogates, and those responsible for the payment of care. Data from these perspectives include their needs and expectations to help design processes and the degree to which these needs and expectation were met to identify areas for improvement. Also, data are collected from these perspectives in relation to relevant dimensions of performance. Staff feedback is elicited through a regular, planned process.

EXAMPLES OF IMPLEMENTATION

1. A hospital designs and implements a pediatric intensive care unit. The staff's assessment includes the need for this service in their organization and community; the needs and expectations of patients who will be treated in the unit and those of their parents; and the expectations of the staff who will work in the unit. From the data collected, a series of design specifications is built into the plans related to the physical facility, the resources (human, technical, and so on), and the care processes. During the new unit's first six months of operation, data are collected as to how well these patient, parent, and staff needs and expectations were met. When not met, improvement strategies are developed and tested.

2. The organization's leaders, in collaboration with staff, identify from their monitoring a number of significant improvement opportunities. Since the opportunities are all resource intensive, the leaders need to set priorities for what is most important and should be accomplished first. To assist in setting the priorities, patients, community residents, staff, and local businesses are surveyed as to their needs and expectations regarding several of the dimensions of performance. The data from this survey are used by the leaders in setting the year's improvement priorities.

EXAMPLES OF EVIDENCE OF PERFORMANCE
- Discussions with patients and staff
- Review of data on needs and expectations of patients, staff, and others
- Review of design and improvement activities

PI.3.4 The organization measures the performance of processes in all the patient care and organizational functions identified in this Manual.

PI.3.4.1 Processes that are measured on a continuing basis include those that

PI.3.4.1.1 affect a large percentage of patients; and/or

PI.3.4.1.2 place patients at serious risk if not performed well, or performed when not indicated, or not performed when indicated; and/or

PI.3.4.1.3 have been or are likely to be problem prone.

INTENT OF PI.3.4 THROUGH PI.3.4.1.3
Because the functions and processes identified in this *Manual* are important to patient outcomes, their performance is measured. Within those functions, processes of particular importance are those that affect a large percentage of patients, place patients at risk, and/or are problem prone. These processes are given priority and are measured on a continuing basis. These processes include those related to surgical and other invasive procedures, the use of medication, and the use of blood and blood components, as applicable.

EXAMPLES OF IMPLEMENTATION
1. A hospital's quality council identified all its important functions related to patient care and organization management. The list included those functions within Section 1 and Section 2 of this *Manual* as well as some additional processes. The council formed small cross-organizational work groups to

flowchart each function and identify the processes and activities within that function that are volume, risk, and problem related. They then designed an organizationwide measurement system that included measurement processes traditionally related to the medical staff (surgery, drugs, blood). Each function or process was assigned to a team representative of the involved or affected departments, disciplines, and individuals. These teams measured the process, tested incremental improvements, and recommended these improvements to relevant department heads or the quality council.

2. The hospital quality improvement department developed a comprehensive profile of all the measurement activities currently used by the organization. They grouped these activities according to the important functions identified by this *Manual.* Small cross-organizational work groups reviewed the measurement activities already being used for a function and consolidated and refined them as necessary. They also identified for future development needed measures for high-risk, high-volume, or problem-prone processes. The quality improvement department developed a plan for facilitating appropriate cross-organizational involvement in the existing measurement of functions and processes and for assisting in the development of measures for other functions.

EXAMPLES OF EVIDENCE OF PERFORMANCE
- Discussions with the organization's leaders, quality/performance improvement staff, work group/team leaders and members
- Meeting minutes
- Strategic, quality, and other planning documents

INTENT OF PI.3.4.2 AND PI.3.4.2.1
Surgical and other invasive procedures are important diagnostic and therapeutic mechanisms, but they often pose considerable risk to the patient. Invasive procedures include, for example, percutaneous aspirations and biopsies, and cardiac and vascular catheterization. If performed when not indicated, surgical and other invasive procedures often expose the patient to substantial,

unnecessary risk. Failure to perform them when indicated may substantially decrease the likelihood of a positive outcome for the patient. Whenever performed, if not performed well, they can expose the patient to the risk of avoidable complications and/or less than optimal benefit. Even when the procedures are performed well, the risk of certain complications may be unavoidable. For these reasons, surgical and other invasive procedures historically have been given special attention in reviewing and improving diagnostic and therapeutic interventions.

The outcome of a surgical or invasive procedure is influenced by the performance of all processes leading to the performance of a particular procedure, as well as the performance of the procedure itself and the monitoring of the patient during and after the procedure. Systematic measurement of processes provides objective information on their performance and identifies areas for possible improvement.

The selection and performance of surgical and other invasive procedures are dependent on the knowledge, judgment, and skills of the practitioner (for example, surgeon, gastroenterologist, cardiologist). However, patient outcomes from performed procedures are dependent also on other factors, such as the laboratory's performance, equipment selection and maintenance, the operating room team (including the anesthesiologist, surgical assistants, operating room nurses, technicians, and so on), and the recovery room procedures.

Historically, surgical case review has focused almost exclusively on the practitioner's knowledge, judgment, and skills, possibly overlooking opportunities for improvement in these other aspects of patient care. For this reason, the standards state that the review activities' results are to be used primarily to study and improve processes involved in selecting and performing surgical and other invasive procedures, thus intentionally broadening the scope of what is studied and improved.

Therefore, these standards require reviewing processes as well as procedures to improve their selection (appropriateness), performance (effectiveness), and outcomes. Although all individuals and professions involved in providing such services are responsible for this review, the medical staff plays a central role and is responsible when the review focuses on the performance of a licensed independent practitioner with clinical privileges.

Any procedure can be reviewed in either or both of the following ways: screening or intensive assessment. Screening refers to the application of predetermined criteria, such as indicators, to individual patient cases to determine whether that case or group of cases should be more intensively assessed. These screening criteria may apply to one specific category of procedure, such as the indications for thyroid surgery, or may apply to a number of categories of procedures, such as surgical infection rates or unscheduled return to the operating room. Such multicategory screening criteria, when very broad in scope, are sometimes referred to as generic screens.

The second type of review is intensive assessment, in which a specific case or group of cases is reviewed intensively. Statistical techniques may be used to uncover patterns or trends in a group of cases, and peers may assess practitioners' knowledge, judgment, and skills. This intensive assessment is often initiated because the screening criteria have identified cases that need further assessment. Sentinel events require timely intensive assessment for every occurrence. However, intensive assessment may also be initiated at other times, such as in response to questions raised by a patient, practitioner, or major insurer. The intensive assessment itself may lead to establishing new screening criteria or initiating screening for a category of procedure not previously encompassed by the review activities.

Both screening and intensively assessing a particular category of procedure must include an adequate number of cases to accomplish the purpose of the review. For low-volume procedures, usually every case must be screened or intensively assessed. High-volume procedures can be sampled; that is, the screening criteria can be applied to a sample of cases (for example, every third), or a sample of cases can be intensively assessed. However, even for high-volume procedures, it is often initially necessary to review every case (either screening or intensive assessment) to establish a baseline so appropriate sampling techniques can be chosen. The medical staff or group undertaking the review should thus carefully decide whether to start sampling initially.

When high-volume cases are sampled, an appropriate sample size must be determined and used. Surveyors will inquire about the sample's rationale and adequacy if it is less than 5% of the average number of cases occurring periodically (not less than quarterly) or 30 cases in that period of time (whichever is larger). The surveyor will use the following guidelines to determine when further inquiry is needed:

- If the average number of cases per quarter is more than 600, at least 5% of cases are reviewed; and
- If the average number of cases per quarter is fewer than 600, at least 30 cases are reviewed.

EXAMPLES OF EVIDENCE OF PERFORMANCE

- Discussions with leaders
- Plans for review
- Documentation of reviews
- Meeting minutes

PI.3.4.2.2 Processes measured encompass at least those related to the use of medications, including (1) prescribing/ ordering medication, (2) preparation and dispensing, (3) administration, and (4) monitoring the medications' effects on patients;

INTENT OF PI.3.4.2.2

Medication is an important component in treating many diseases—in many cases it is the most important intervention.

Yet most medications have potentially serious risks associated with their use, such as common short-term side effects, idiosyncratic responses, medication-medication interactions, food-medication interactions, and side effects associated with long-term use and toxic levels. Thus, if a medication is not administered when needed, a patient may not achieve the full benefits of therapy, but when administered when not needed, the patient may experience unnecessary risks. Likewise, when administered correctly, certain risks (for example, common side effects) may be present, and when administered incorrectly, these risks may be magnified and new risks, such as medication-medication interactions, introduced. For these reasons, medication usage has historically been given special attention when reviewing and improving diagnostic and therapeutic interventions.

A hospital uses so many medications that they cannot all be routinely assessed. Therefore, priorities are set for the ongoing assessment of medication use. These priorities are based on the number of patients affected by a medication use (that is, the frequency of an order for medication); the significance, especially the degree of risk, of the medication use for an individual patient; and the degree to which use of the medication is known or suspected to be problem prone. Medication assessment priorities can also be based on priorities established for studying and improving the treatment of a specific disease for which medication is integral to treatment, such as using antibiotics in treating pneumonia. Whichever of these reasons, or combination thereof, guides the choice of medication for review, the review itself encompasses the full set of processes (prescribing/ordering, preparing and dispensing, administration, and monitoring the effects on patients) and does not focus primarily on the practitioners' knowledge, judgment, and skill; doing the latter misses many opportunities to improve medication use.

Therefore, these standards require assessing the processes of medication use to improve their appropriateness and effectiveness. The assessment uses predetermined criteria to review the use of selected medications. These criteria can screen use to identify cases, or groups of cases, requiring more intensive assessment. Predetermined criteria can also more intensively assess specific cases, or groups of cases, to identify improvement opportunities. When medications are used in high volume, a sample of the medication under review may be screened or intensively assessed rather than reviewing every case of use.

The appropriate and effective use of medications is dependent on many factors, such as the physician's knowledge, judgment, and skill in ordering medications; the pharmacy's preparation and dispensing of medications; the transmittal of medication orders; the transport of medication in the hospital; the nurse's administration of medications; and the physician's and nurse's monitoring of medications' effects. Therefore, medication use is assessed in a cross-departmental, cross-discipline cooperative effort by the pharmacy department, nursing, management and administrative staff, and others, as required. The medical staff is responsible for the assessment when it focuses on the performance of a licensed independent practitioner with clinical privileges.

EXAMPLES OF EVIDENCE OF PERFORMANCE
- Discussions with leaders
- Plans for review
- Documentation of ongoing reviews
- Meeting minutes

INTENT OF PI.3.4.2.3
The administration of blood and blood components is often a significant component of care for individual patients with respect to therapeutic potential and risk. If administered when not indicated, blood or blood components may expose the patient to substantial unnecessary risk, such as hepatitis. Failure to administer them when indicated may substantially decrease the likelihood of a positive outcome for the patient. When used incorrectly, blood and blood components can also expose the patient to the risk of avoidable complications and/or less than optimal benefit. Even when used correctly, the risk of certain complications may be unavoidable. For these reasons, the use of blood and blood components has historically been given special attention when reviewing and improving diagnostic and therapeutic interventions.

Patient outcomes from the use of blood and blood components are dependent on factors, such as the laboratory transfusion service's performance, equipment selection and maintenance, the ordering physician's knowledge, judgment, and skill, and the nursing staff's performance. Historically, blood usage review has focused on the ordering physician's knowledge, judgment, and skill, overlooking improvement opportunities in these other aspects of patient care.

Therefore, these standards require reviewing several processes related to the use of blood and blood components to improve their appropriateness and effectiveness. All disciplines and departments involved in reviewing the use of blood and blood components are responsible for the review, including, for example, the medical staff, the transfusion service, a number of departments/services that use blood and blood components, or a hospitalwide committee.

Any blood or blood product can be reviewed by screening and/or intensive assessment. Screening refers to the application of predetermined criteria, such as indicators used in the measurement and assessment process, to individual patient cases in which blood or a blood component has been administered to determine whether that case, or group of cases, should be more intensively assessed. These screening criteria can apply to one specific category of blood or blood component, such as the indications for use of platelet concentrate, or to a number of categories of blood or blood components, such as transfusion reactions.

The second type of review is intensive assessment, in which a specific case, or group of cases, is reviewed intensively. Statistical techniques may be used to uncover patterns or trends in a group of cases. When the review focuses on the performance of a licensed independent practitioner with clinical privileges, the medical staff is responsible. This intensive assessment is often initiated because the screening criteria have identified cases needing further assessment. However, intensive assessment may also be initiated at other times, such as in response to questions raised by a patient, practitioner, or major insurer. The intensive assessment itself may lead to establishing new screening criteria for a category of blood or blood components.

Whether screening or intensively assessing a particular category of blood or blood components, the organization includes an adequate number of cases to accomplish the review's purpose. For components used in low volume, usually every case must be screened or intensively assessed. For high-volume blood or blood components, it is often appropriate to sample its use; that is, the screening criteria can be applied to a sample of cases (for example, every third), or a sample of cases can be intensively assessed. However, even for blood or blood components used in high volume, it is often initially necessary to review every case (either by screening or intensive assessment) to establish a baseline, so appropriate sampling techniques can be chosen. The medical staff or group undertaking the review should carefully decide whether to start sampling initially.

When high-volume cases are sampled, an appropriate sample size is determined and used. Surveyors will inquire about the sample's rationale and adequacy if it is less than 5% of the average number of cases occurring periodically (not less than quarterly) or 30 cases in that period of time (whichever is larger). The surveyor will use the following guidelines to determine when further inquiry is needed:

- If the average number of cases per quarter is more than 600, at least 5% of cases are reviewed; and
- If the average number of cases per quarter is fewer than 600, at least 30 cases are reviewed.

By definition, sentinel events are reviewed in a timely manner each and every time they occur.

EXAMPLES OF EVIDENCE OF PERFORMANCE
- Discussion with leaders
- Plans for review
- Documentation of ongoing reviews
- Meeting minutes

PI.3.4.2.4 [Processes measured encompass at least] those related to determining the appropriateness of admissions and continued hospitalization (that is, utilization review activities).

INTENT OF PI.3.4.2.4
Data support any process used to review the appropriateness of admissions and the clinical necessity of continued stay in the organization. The data support concurrent and periodic review processes. Data that may be needed to support the review process

can relate to, for example, age/disability groups, diagnoses, problems, levels of care, and treatment.

EXAMPLES OF EVIDENCE OF PERFORMANCE
- Plans for utilization review
- Meeting minutes
- Reports
- Patient medical records

PI.3.5 The organization collects data about

PI.3.5.1 autopsy results,

PI.3.5.2 risk management activities, and

PI.3.5.3 quality control activities in at least the following areas:

PI.3.5.3.1 Clinical laboratory services,

PI.3.5.3.2 Diagnostic radiology services,

PI.3.5.3.3 Dietetic services,

PI.3.5.3.4 Nuclear medicine services, and

PI.3.5.3.5 Radiation oncology services.

INTENT OF PI.3.5 THROUGH PI.3.5.3.5
Autopsies, risk management, and quality control have the potential to provide relevant and important information for systematic and organizationwide improvement. Data collection for these activities has frequently not been guided by clear assessment criteria or has not been shared with those responsible for performance improvement activities because the data were considered confidential. Many different departments/services, disciplines, and individuals must cooperate to integrate the data collection for

these activities into the overall framework for data collection.

This cooperation is especially important for risk management functions. There are operational links between the risk management functions and the clinical aspects of patient care, patient safety, and performance improvement. Those individuals responsible for improving processes need access to existing information from risk management activities that may help identify opportunities to improve those processes.

EXAMPLES OF EVIDENCE OF PERFORMANCE

- Discussions with leaders
- Plans for data collection
- Committees' reports and minutes

Assess

Based on the objective measurement of the performance of existing processes and outcomes, an organization can, by interpreting the collected data, answer questions such as

- What is our current level of performance and the stability of our current processes?
- Are there areas that could be improved?
- Was a strategy to stabilize or improve performance effective?
- Were design specifications of new processes met?

The frame of reference for interpreting the collected data can be internal comparisons over time; comparison to state-of-the-art sources, such as standards (accreditation standards) and practice guidelines (parameters); and/or comparison with the performance of similar processes and outcomes in other organizations (reference/comparative databases).

When designing new processes or redesigning existing processes, other data, such as law and regulatory requirements, are also essential design factors.

Conclusions from measurement about the need for more intensive measurement and assessment can be drawn by interpreting the data and by comparison to preestablished criteria, a single sentinel event, control limits, or the review of all occurrences.

When operating well, the assessment process is interdisciplinary and interdepartmental as appropriate for the process and/or outcome under review. The medical staff, using peer review, is responsible for the assessment process when an individual licensed independent practitioner's performance is the focus.

PI.4 The organization has a systematic process to assess collected data in order to determine
- *whether design specifications for new processes were met;*
- *the level of performance and stability of important existing processes;*
- *priorities for possible improvement of existing processes;*
- *actions to improve the performance of processes; and*
- *whether changes in the processes resulted in improvement.*

INTENT OF PI.4

Data essential to addressing performance questions posed in advance are collected, and the questions are clearly identified for assessing that data.

This systematic assessment framework applies to a variety of assessment questions in the organization and, as frequently as possible, it assesses the data against predetermined performance expectations, design specifications, or other applicable criteria.

EXAMPLE OF IMPLEMENTATION

An organization's new ambulatory care facility has been in operation for six months. Considerable resources have been directed toward assessing a variety of questions: Did the patients/families like the facility and services (were their needs and expectations met)? Did the outcomes of the care processes meet expectations (predetermined criteria), and were they stable even though the volume of patients grew rapidly (only "common cause" variation)? Were the intervention improvement strategies at the patient registration desk successful (unacceptable variation in wait times now acceptable)? Were there other opportunities to improve that had not been acted on yet (staff and other specifications not met)?

The organization instructed all staff involved in this assessment phase how to use performance improvement tools, such as control charts, and coached them through a uniform process to assess the data they collected.

EXAMPLES OF EVIDENCE OF PERFORMANCE
- Discussions with leaders and improvement teams
- Records of meetings
- Reports of assessment conclusions and strategies
- Education/training records

PI.4.1 The assessment process includes

PI.4.1.1 using statistical quality control techniques, as appropriate.

INTENT OF PI.4.1 AND PI.4.1.1
An understanding of statistical quality control techniques and variation is essential for an effective assessment process. Together they focus the organization's attention and resources on those processes and outcomes for which more intensive assessment would be most beneficial. That level of assessment is initiated by comparison with self (levels/patterns/trends), with others (reference databases), with standards (practice guidelines), and with best practices (improve already good performance to the leaders' level).

EXAMPLE OF IMPLEMENTATION
An operating room shortage was perceived as a major problem for a busy surgical suite in a 300-bed community hospital. Before recommending that the suite be enlarged by six more operating rooms, a team was selected to measure current use. The team chose from a number of issues the turnaround time between cases, defined as the period of time from the end of anesthesia on a case to the start of anesthesia on the next case. The team measured turnaround time for 4 months and used statistical quality control techniques to look at the variation in times over that period. A number of strategies were tested, and over the next few months, mean turnaround time was reduced from 92 minutes

to 48 minutes, and the variation evident between shifts was reduced to what was considered acceptable common-cause levels.

EXAMPLES OF EVIDENCE OF PERFORMANCE

- Discussions with leaders and quality improvement staff and teams
- Reports and minutes
- Improvement strategies and plans

INTENT OF PI.4.1.2 THROUGH PI.4.1.2.3

Assessment questions can be answered from two perspectives: What is the performance of a process compared internally over time, and what is the performance of the process compared to external sources of information related to the process (performance being measured using process and outcome measures)?

Information from external sources is as up-to-date as possible, such as recent scientific, clinical, and management literature, well-formulated practice guidelines or parameters, reference databases, and standards that benefit from periodic review and revision.

Note: The goal of an organization is to develop an assessment process that incorporates four basic comparisons: with self, with others, with standards, and with best practices.

To move organizations toward this goal, the compliance expectations for organizations will be increased incrementally over the next few years. This also recognizes that it may take a few years for an organization's information management capabilities to be in line with the expectation set by this standard.

Most organizations are currently able, or will be able in a short time, to obtain and use information from such reference sources as the literature and practice guidelines/parameters. The initial expectation for these sources will thus be high.

Few organizations currently participate in external reference databases or will in a short time be able to do so fully. The initial expectation for these sources will be modest.

The reference databases to which the standards refer are those designed to accept data from the organization and provide feedback on the organization's performance compared to that of other organizations and in a form useful to the organization (for example, adjusted for differences in patient population).

In 1994, organizations will be expected to contribute to one such external reference database (in addition to data provided to the Health Care Financing Administration as part of routine reporting) in assessing their performance. Examples of such databases are those operated by multihospital systems, the Department of Veterans Affairs, the Joint Commission's indicator monitoring system, and other multihospital, state, and/or regional databases.

The Joint Commission's indicator monitoring system will be operational in 1994 and 1995 for organizations to participate in this database on a voluntary basis. Whenthe system is integrated into the accreditation process, participation will be mandatory for all hospitals seeking accreditation.

EXAMPLES OF EVIDENCE OF PERFORMANCE
- Discussions with leaders, information service staff, and performance improvement teams
- Reports and minutes
- Improvement plans and strategies
- Assessment conclusions/reports

PI.4.1.3 [The assessment process includes] intensive assessment when undesirable variation in performance may have occurred or is occurring. Such intensive assessments are initiated

PI.4.1.3.1 by important single events and by absolute levels and/or patterns/trends that significantly and undesirably vary from those expected, based on appropriate statistical analysis;

PI.4.1.3.2 when the organization's performance significantly and undesirably varies from that of other organizations;

PI.4.1.3.3 when the organization's performance significantly and undesirably varies from recognized standards;

PI.4.1.3.4 when the organization wishes to improve already good performance;

INTENT OF PI.4.1.3 THROUGH PI.4.1.3.4
When an organization begins to compare its performance over time as described in PI.4.1.2 through PI.4.1.2.3, intensive assessment is appropriate at times. Understanding variation is essential to this activity. Only then can the organization initiate appropriate and timely further assessment to return or bring performance to desired levels of stability.

EXAMPLE OF IMPLEMENTATION

A metropolitan hospital with a busy emergency department has been measuring the timeliness and appropriateness (two dimensions of performance) of the patient assessment process in the emergency department. Data have been collected for a variety of measures for over 6 months. A team consisting of a nurse, an emergency physician, a radiologist, and an administrator has been reviewing the data each month. Although there has not been a single sentinel event to trigger intensive assessment, the team has noticed a slowly lengthening turnaround time for diagnostic tests. Also, a comparison with a similar hospital in another part of the city indicates that wait time and total time in the emergency unit are 20% higher than those of the similar organization. Recently, the emergency physician obtained the practice guidelines for treating chest pain and would like to implement the guidelines. Based on all this, the team decides to intensively assess the related processes and outcomes before developing a set of priority strategies for improvement.

EXAMPLES OF EVIDENCE OF PERFORMANCE

- Discussions with leaders, information service staff, and performance improvement teams
- Assessment conclusions/reports

PI.4.1.3.5 [The assessment process includes intensive assessment when undesirable variation in performance may have occurred or is occurring. Such intensive assessments are initiated] in response to all major discrepancies, or patterns of discrepancies, between preoperative and postoperative (including pathologic) diagnoses, including those identified during the pathologic review of specimens removed during surgical or invasive procedures;

PI.4.1.3.6 by all confirmed transfusion reactions; and

PI.4.1.3.7 by all significant adverse drug reactions.

INTENT OF PI.4.1.3.5 THROUGH PI.4.1.3.7

When measuring surgical and other invasive procedures (PI.3.4.2.1), medication use (PI.3.4.2.2), and use of blood and blood components (PI.3.4.2.3), *three events* always elicit further assessment: major discrepancies between preoperative and postoperative diagnoses, confirmed transfusion reactions, and significant adverse drug reactions.

EXAMPLES OF EVIDENCE OF PERFORMANCE

* Reports of assessment conclusions
* Meeting minutes
* Pathology reports

PI.4.2 When the findings of the assessment process are relevant to an individual's performance,

PI.4.2.1 the medical staff is responsible for determining their use in peer review and/or the periodic evaluations of a licensed independent practitioner's competence, in accordance with the standards on renewing/revising clinical privileges delineated in the "Medical Staff" chapter; and/or

PI.4.2.2 the department/service director is responsible for determining the competence of individuals who are not licensed independent practitioners, in accordance with standard LD.2.1.2.5.

INTENT OF PI.4.2 THROUGH PI.4.2.2

Data assessment is a systematic process to determine performance in relation to the design specifications of processes, to determine the level of functioning of processes, to identify opportunities for improvement, and to review outcomes in relation to expectations. Each of these determinations can also result in the identification of an individual's performance as a relevant factor. When such an initial determination has been made, steps for further review, final recommendation, and any action and follow-up are required.

Such steps are identified in the "Medical Staff" chapter in 1994 in relation to licensed independent practitioners and the "Management of Human Resources" chapter in 1995 for others (see GB.1.14 in 1994). In each case, the director of the relevant department/service is responsible for seeing that the steps are followed, that the individual's personnel or credentials file contains the findings, and that those findings, when relevant, are used in reappraising the individual.

EXAMPLES OF IMPLEMENTATION

1. A special care cardiac unit decided to assess intensively its medication use in an effort to reduce the adverse drug reaction rate below the current level that was stable at acceptable or predictable levels. The data from the intensive assessment indicated a higher rate of significant adverse drug reactions during one particular weekend shift and when certain medications were prescribed by one particular medical staff member. The team overseeing this improvement effort continued assessing the data related to the shift differences and provided the director of the medical staff member's department with data that called that individual's performance into question. The director initiated a peer review for the individual's performance. The findings were used in the periodic evaluation process for renewing privileges as described in the "Medical Staff" chapter.

2. A hospital's medical-surgical unit was intensively assessing the timeliness of consultation requests/responses because there appeared to be undesirable variation by shift and by day of the week. The assessment's results indicated that one unit clerk was not processing the consultation requests properly. The medical department director and the human resources director reviewed the data, created a retraining program for the one staff member, and continued to monitor timeliness to provide evidence that the staff member was properly processing requests and that undesirable variation was reduced.

EXAMPLES OF EVIDENCE OF PERFORMANCE

• Reports of assessment activities

- Meeting minutes
- Personnel and credentials files

Improve

Improving the performance of existing processes and improving outcomes are desirable results of an organizationwide performance improvement function. This can be accomplished as independent incremental improvements or as a part of a series of incremental improvements to redesign a process effectively.

Most organizations identify more opportunities to improve than can be acted on; thus, priorities are set. Criteria are helpful in setting priorities and could include the relation of the potential improvement to the important functions described in this *Manual*; those criteria identified in this chapter for use in selecting processes to measure; and the expected impact on the dimensions of performance.

Once the decision has been made to implement an improvement strategy or test a strategy, the relevant departments and disciplines are involved, and a performance measure(s) is selected against which to assess the success of the actions taken. On occasion the actions taken may modify an individual's clinical privileges or job assignment.

PI.5 The organization systematically improves its performance by improving existing processes.

INTENT OF PI.5

When an existing process is to be redesigned or the organization decides to act on an opportunity for incremental improvement in an existing process, the organization has a systematic approach. A systematic approach is one that includes identifying a potential improvement, testing the strategy for change, assessing data from the test to determine if the change produced improved performance, and implementing the improvement strategy systemwide. The Joint Commission's ten-step process is one such approach; however, there are many others that follow a similar scientific inquiry method to provide a similar systematic process for improvement. What works best for an organization is established as the singular approach to be used by all its improvement teams. A singular approach facilitates the data sharing required in the "Management of Information" chapter of this *Manual.*

EXAMPLE OF IMPLEMENTATION

A small community hospital's quality council has been reviewing the organization's process improvement approaches. Whereas several departments are using the Joint Commission's ten-step process, a few departments involved in cross-departmental improvements have been using a modified FOCUS-PDCA approach. The quality council arranged a seminar on process-improvement approaches that resulted in the appointment of a cross-departmental work group to recommend a single approach for the hospital. The work group recommended a further modified FOCUS-PDCA approach and that the approach be renamed with the hospital's name to increase ownership and reduce confusion. All quality improvement teams were then retrained in the uniform approach.

EXAMPLES OF EVIDENCE OF PERFORMANCE

- Discussions with leaders, performance improvement staff, and improvement teams
- Planning documents
- Training materials
- Reports and meeting minutes

PI.5.1 Existing processes are improved when an organization decides to act on an opportunity for improvement or when the measurement of an existing process identifies that an undesirable change in performance may have occurred or is occurring.

PI.5.1.1 These decisions consider

PI.5.1.1.1 opportunities to improve processes within the important functions described in this **Manual;**

PI.5.1.1.2 the factors listed in PI.3.3 through PI.3.5.3.5;

PI.5.1.1.3 the resources required to make the improvement; and

PI.5.1.1.4 the organization's mission and priorities.

INTENT OF PI.5.1 THROUGH PI.5.1.1.4

The organization's leaders are responsible for setting priorities for improvement, either incrementally improving an already well-operating process or reducing variation or eliminating undesirable change in existing processes. This setting of priorities is guided by accepted criteria. Those criteria include the important functions described in this *Manual* and the measurement factors identified in PI.3.3 through PI.3.5.3.5; the criteria also consider the resources required to make the improvement and how the improvement will relate to the organization's "mission critical" activities.

EXAMPLE OF IMPLEMENTATION

A 250-bed urban hospital has a very active emergency department with a high percentage of admissions coming through that department. Patient assessment is very slow due to the diagnostic radiology equipment's location, the equipment's age, and the clinical laboratory's location. Patients are unhappy, staff cannot be efficient, and frequently a patient is admitted prior to the completion of all assessments. Although patient assessment in the emergency department is the highest-priority organizationwide improvement, all parts of the organization will continue to carry out the important task of keeping current processes stable and making incremental improvements in those processes.

EXAMPLES OF EVIDENCE OF PERFORMANCE

- Discussions with leaders and improvement staff
- Plans and strategies for improvement
- Meeting minutes
- Established criteria for priority setting

PI.5.2 *The design or improvement activities*

PI.5.2.1 *specifically consider the expected impact of the design or improvement on the relevant dimensions of performance;*

PI.5.2.2 *set performance expectations for the design or improvement of the processes;*

PI.5.2.3 *include adopting, adapting, or creating measures of the performance; and*

PI.5.2.4 *involve those individuals, professions, and departments/services closest to the design or improvement activity.*

INTENT OF PI.5.2 THROUGH PI.5.2.4

Before acting on a design or improvement activity, the organization asks four questions:

- What dimension(s) of performance will be most affected by the change, and is there an interaction between dimensions that must be considered (for example, when a service's availability is increased, the process' efficiency may decline)?
- How do we expect/want the improved process to perform?
- How will we measure that the process is actually performing at the level we expect/want?
- Who is closest to this process and thus should own or be involved in the improvement activity?

These basic operational questions are fundamental to implementing a design or improvement activity. Additional design or improvement specifications include regulatory requirements and accreditation decisions and recommendations.

EXAMPLE OF IMPLEMENTATION

Over the years, a small suburban hospital computerized many activities, such as billing, appointments, clinical laboratory, and purchasing. These systems were planned and implemented independently and thus are not connected in a planned manner. A team of individuals from information services, medical records, clinical laboratories, library services, and management studied how the hospital manages patient care information and how it can improve. From a comprehensive needs assessment, they prepared a set of performance expectations for a reconstituted and integrated system. One of the team's concerns was that during the two-year transition phase, as access to information increased, the timeliness for some information and for some users would decrease. They selected information access and timeliness measures to monitor this potential problem. The implementation plan had four phases that would affect different clinical areas in each phase. For each phase, a user team was formed, composed of the individuals who would manage and use the system when implemented. These user teams were educated in process improvement   and eventually trained the remaining staff.

EXAMPLES OF EVIDENCE OF PERFORMANCE
- Discussion with leaders and improvement staff
- Plans, reports, and minutes

PI.5.3 When action is taken to improve a process,

PI.5.3.1 the action may be tested on a trial basis;

PI.5.3.1.1 When the initial action is not effective, a new action is planned and tested.

PI.5.3.2 the action's effect is assessed; and

PI.5.3.3 successful actions are implemented.

INTENT OF PI.5.3 THROUGH PI.5.3.3
Once performance expectations have been established and performance measures identified, the design or improvement activity is tested or implemented, even if that means the variation or other undesirable change continues during the test period.

When the action is assessed as ineffective, a new action is planned and tested. Finally, when the assessment shows the action to be successful, it is implemented where appropriate.

EXAMPLE OF IMPLEMENTATION

A performance improvement team at a medium-sized rural hospital has been reviewing the process of medication prescribing/ordering. Measurement data reveal a pattern of unacceptable variation in timeliness and accuracy; therefore, a plan of action has been prepared. Because the hospital is not able to implement an electronic process, it has considerably revised the work forms, training of staff, transport process, and verification process. The staff on the general medicine unit were eager to test the new processes, and a three-month trial period was started. They continued to measure timeliness and accuracy and found that all but one of the new processes resulted in improvement; this process was redesigned and retested, resulting in improvement. All the new processes for prescribing/ordering were then implemented on a unit-by-unit basis.

EXAMPLES OF EVIDENCE OF PERFORMANCE

- Discussion with improvement staff and teams
- Reports, records, and minutes
- Assessment data
- Improvement plans

PI.5.4 Action is directed primarily at improving processes.

PI.5.4.1 Pursuant to PI.4.2, when improvement activities lead to a determination that an individual has performance problems that he/she is unable or unwilling to improve, his/her clinical privileges or job assignment is modified (in accordance with the standards in this **Manual [AMH, Vol I]** *on renewing/revising clinical privileges in the "Medical Staff" chapter and on determining competence in GB.1.14 in 1994 and in the "Management of Human Re-*

*sources" chapter in 1995), as indicated, or some other appro-
priate action is taken.*

INTENT OF PI.5.4 AND PI.5.4.1

Individual performance information is assessed through the
processes described in PI.4.2. Occasionally, however, individual
performance issues are identified when an improvement strategy
is implemented.

No matter when an individual's performance is an issue, when
confirmed through the processes described in PI.4.2, the individual
is given not only sufficient opportunity to change, but also education
to bring his/her performance to the desired level. If the individual's
performance does not improve, then other appropriate actions are
taken, such as an assignment change. Whatever action is taken, it
conforms to established policy and protocol as identified in the
"Medical Staff" chapter in 1994, GB.1.14 in 1994, and/or the "Management of Human Resources" chapter in 1995.

EXAMPLES OF IMPLEMENTATION

1. In one organization, the introduction of a computerized
    tracking system significantly improved the organizationwide
    program for measuring infections in terms of timeliness and
    accuracy. The individual responsible for tracking was using a
    paper-and-pencil process and, in consultation with the
    department/service director, chose not to gain the computer
    skills needed for the new process. The individual requested to
    transfer to another department where his/her skills were
    appropriate and the processes were not computerized.
2. The measurement of outcomes for total hip replacement led
    the Department of Surgery at an organization to conclude that
    variation in outcomes could be significantly reduced if only
    two types of prostheses were used rather than the five types
    currently preferred by the surgeons. Two surgeons who
    initially preferred another type of prosthesis improved their
    skills related to the selected prostheses; therefore, their clinical
    privileges were not changed. However, one surgeon chose not

to improve his/her skills but continued to use a prosthesis of his/her choice at another hospital. That surgeon's clinical privileges were modified for that particular procedure in accordance with medical staff established policy.

EXAMPLES OF EVIDENCE OF PERFORMANCE

- Discussion with leaders, improvement staff and teams, and individuals
- Reports
- Meeting minutes
- Credentials and personnel files

Appendix C

This appendix contains three sections: (1) the indicators selected for the Joint Commission's indicator monitoring system, which began operation in 1994; (2) the indicators currently undergoing beta testing in the field; and (3) other indicators recommended by the Joint Commission's Board of Commissioners for hospitals' internal use.

1994 INDICATOR MONITORING SYSTEM INDICATORS

Although some Joint Commission indicator sets continue progressing through a multiyear testing phase, the anesthesia and obstetrical care indicator sets have completed this process. Based on the results of this testing and recommendations from expert task forces, the Board of Commissioners has approved the indicators in this section for the indicator monitoring system in which hospitals may participate on an optional basis.

The following indicators are included in the indicator monitoring system in 1994.*

1. **Numerator:** Patients developing a central nervous system (CNS) complication within two postprocedure days of procedures involving anesthesia* administration.

---

*For the indicators related to anesthesia care, the population of interest includes all patients undergoing surgical procedures involving anesthesia. Anesthesia is defined as the administration (in any setting, for any purpose, by any route) of general, spinal, or other major regional anesthesia or sedation (with or without analgesia) for which there is a reasonable expectation that, in the manner used, the sedation/analgesia will result in the loss of protective reflexes for a significant percentage of a group of patients.

Denominator: All patients undergoing surgical procedures involving anesthesia administration and having an inpatient stay.

2. **Numerator:** Patients developing a peripheral neurologic deficit within two postprocedure days of procedures involving anesthesia administration.

   Denominator: All patients undergoing surgical procedures involving anesthesia administration and having an inpatient stay.

3. **Numerator:** Patients developing an acute myocardial infarction (AMI) within two postprocedure days of procedures involving anesthesia administration.

   Denominator: All patients undergoing surgical procedures involving anesthesia administration and having an inpatient stay.

4. **Numerator:** Patients with a cardiac arrest within two postprocedure days of procedures involving anesthesia administration.

   Denominator: All patients undergoing surgical procedures involving anesthesia administration and having an inpatient stay.

5. **Numerator:** Intrahospital mortality of patients within two postprocedure days of procedures involving anesthesia administration.

   Denominator: All patients undergoing surgical procedures

For the indicators related to anesthesia care, the population of interest includes all patients undergoing surgical procedures involving anesthesia. Anesthesia is defined as the administration (in any setting, for any purpose, by any route) of general, spinal, or other major regional anesthesia or sedation (with or without analgesia) for which there is a reasonable expectation that, in the manner used, the sedation/analgesia will result in the loss of protective reflexes for a significant percentage of a group of patients.

involving anesthesia administration and having an inpatient stay.

6. **Numerator:** Patients delivered by cesarean section.

   Denominator: All deliveries.

7. **Numerator:** Patients with vaginal birth after cesarean section (VBAC).

   Denominator: Patients delivered with a history of previous cesarean section.

8. **Numerator:** Live-born infants with a birthweight less than 2,500 grams.

   Denominator: All live births.

9. **Numerator:** Live-born infants with a birthweight greater than or equal to 2,500 grams, who have at least one of the following: an Apgar score of less than 4 at five minutes, a requirement for admission to the neonatal intensive care unit (NICU) within one day of delivery for greater than 24 hours, a clinically apparent seizure or significant birth trauma

   Denominator: All live-born infants with a birthweight greater than or equal to 2,500 grams.

10. **Numerator:** Live-born infants with a birthweight greater than 1,000 grams and less than 2,500 grams who have an Apgar score of less than 4 at five minutes

    Denominator: All live-born infants with a birthweight greater than 1,000 grams and less than 2,500 grams

INDICATORS CURRENTLY IN BETA TESTING

The following indicators are currently undergoing beta testing as part of the development and testing process for Joint Commission indicators. They are recommended for use by hospitals.*

Cardiovascular Indicators

Cardiovascular Patient Population: The cardiovascular indicators draw from four populations described in the following paragraphs: coronary artery bypass grafts (CABG), percutaneous transluminal coronary angioplasty (PTCA), acute myocardial infarction (MI), and congestive heart failure (CHF)

CABG Patient Population: Patients undergoing CABG excluding those with other cardiac or peripheral vascular surgical procedures performed at the time of the CABG (for example, valve replacement)

CV-1 **Indicator Focus:** Intrahospital mortality as a means of assessing multiple aspects of CABG care
Indicator (Numerator): Intrahospital mortality of patients undergoing isolated CABG procedures, subcategorized by initial or subsequent CABG procedures, emergent or nonemergent clinical status, and postoperative day and intrahospital location of death

CV-2 **Indicator Focus:** Extended postoperative stay as a means of assessing multiple aspects of CABG care
Indicator (Numerator): Patients with prolonged postoperative stay for isolated CABG procedures subcategorized by initial or subsequent CABG procedures, emergent or nonemergent procedures, and the use or nonuse of a circulatory support device

PTCA Patient Population: Patients for whom a PTCA procedure is initiated, regardless of whether a lesion is crossed or dilated

---

The final wording of each indicator in this section may be subject to revision based on the results of further testing.

CV-3 *Indicator Focus:* Intrahospital mortality as a means of assessing multiple aspects of PTCA care
Indicator (Numerator): Intrahospital mortality of patients following PTCA subcategorized by emergent or nonemergent clinical status, postprocedure day, and intrahospital location of death

CV-4 *Indicator Focus:* Specific clinical events as a means of assessing multiple aspects of PTCA care
Indicator (Numerator): Patients undergoing nonemergent PTCA with subsequent occurrence of either an acute MI or CABG procedure within the same hospitalization

CV-5 *Indicator Focus:* Effectiveness of PTCA
Indicator (Numerator): Patients undergoing attempted or completed PTCA during which any lesion attempted is not dilated

MI Patient Population: Patients with a principal diagnosis of acute MI either on hospital discharge, emergency department (ED) transfer to another acute care facility, or death in the ED, and patients who are admitted for an acute MI or to rule out an acute MI

CV-6 *Indicator Focus:* Intrahospital mortality as a means of assessing multiple aspects of acute MI care
Indicator (Numerator): Intrahospital mortality of patients with principal discharge diagnosis of acute MI subcategorized by history of previous infarction, age, and intrahospital location of death

CV-7 *Indicator Focus:* Diagnostic accuracy and resource utilization
Indicator (Numerator): Patients admitted for acute MI, to rule out acute MI, or for unstable angina who have a discharge diagnosis of acute MI subcategorized by admission to an intensive care unit, a monitored bed, or an unmonitored bed

CHF Patient Population: Patients with a discharge diagnosis of CHF with or without specific etiologies

CV-8 **Indicator Focus:** Diagnostic accuracy
Indicator (Numerator): Patients with discharge diagnosis of CHF with documented etiology and chest x-ray substantiation of CHF

CV-9 **Indicator Focus:** Monitoring patients' response to therapy
Indicator (Numerator): Patients with a principal discharge diagnosis of CHF and with at least two determinations of patient weight and of serum sodium, potassium, blood urea nitrogen, and creatinine levels

Oncology Indicators

Oncology Patient Population: Inpatients admitted for initial diagnosis and/or treatment of primary lung, colon, rectal, or female breast cancer

ON-1 **Indicator Focus:** Availability of data for diagnosis and staging
Indicator (Numerator): Surgical pathology consultation reports (pathology reports) containing histological type, tumor size, status of margins, appropriate lymph node examination, assessment of invasion or extension as indicated, and AJCC/pTN classification for patients with resection for primary cancer of the lung, colon/rectum, or female breast

ON-2 **Indicator Focus:** Use of staging by managing physicians
Indicator (Numerator): Patients undergoing treatment for primary cancer of the lung, colon/rectum, or female breast with AJCC stage of tumor designated by a managing physician

ON-3 **Indicator Focus:** Effectiveness of cancer treatment
Indicator (Numerator): Survival of patients with primary

cancer of the lung, colon/rectum, or female breast by stage and histologic type*

ON-4 *Indicator Focus:* Use of tests critical to diagnosis, prognosis, and clinical management
Indicator (Numerator): Female patients with invasive primary breast cancer undergoing initial biopsy or resection of a tumor larger than 1 centimeter in greatest dimension who have presence of estrogen receptor diagnostic analysis results in medical record

ON-5 *Indicator Focus:* Use of multimodal therapy in treatment and follow-up
Indicator (Numerator): Female patients with AJCC Stage II pathologic lymph node positive primary invasive breast cancer treated with systemic adjuvant therapy

ON-6 *Indicator Focus:* Effectiveness of preoperative diagnosis and staging
Indicator (Numerator): Patients with non-small-cell primary lung cancer undergoing thoracotomy with complete surgical resection of tumor

ON-7 *Indicator Focus:* Specific clinical events as a means of assessing multiple aspects of surgical care for lung cancers
Indicator (Numerator): Patients undergoing pulmonary resection for primary lung cancer with postoperative complication of empyema, bronchopleural fistula, reoperation for postoperative bleeding, mechanical ventilation greater than five days postoperatively, or intrahospital death

ON-8 *Indicator Focus:* Comprehensiveness of diagnostic workup
Indicator (Numerator): Patients with resections of primary colorectal cancer whose preoperative evaluation by a managing physician includes examination of the entire

---

* *Efficient mechanisms to obtain postdischarge data will be explored only with a subset of beta-test hospitals. Ability to obtain these data during beta testing is not a requirement of participation.*

colon, liver function tests, chest x-ray, and carcinoemb-
ryonic antigen levels

ON-9 *Indicator Focus:* Documentation of staging, prognosis,
and surgical treatment
Indicator (Numerator): Patients with resection of primary
colorectal cancer whose operative reports include location
of primary tumor, local extent of disease, extent of resection, and assessment of residual abdominal disease

ON-10 *Indicator Focus:* Use of treatment approaches that impact
on quality of life
Indicator (Numerator): Patients with primary rectal cancer
undergoing abdominoperineal resections with 6 centimeters
or more of free distal surgical margin present on specimen,
as documented in surgical pathology gross description

ON-11 *Indicator Focus:* Interdisciplinary treatment and follow-up
Indicator (Numerator): Patients with AJCC Stage II or III
primary rectal cancer with documentation of referral to or
treatment by a radiation or medical oncologist

Trauma Indicators

Trauma Patient Population: Patients with ICD-9-CM diagnostic
code of 800 through 959.9 who either are admitted to the hospital,
die in the emergency department (ED), or are transferred from the
hospital or the ED to another acute care facility, excluding patients
with the following isolated injuries: burns; hip fractures in the
elderly; specified fractures of the face, hand, and foot; and specified
eye wounds

TR-1 *Indicator Focus:* Efficiency of emergency medical services
(EMS)
Indicator (Numerator): Trauma patients with prehospital
EMS scene time greater than 20 minutes

TR-2 *Indicator Focus:* Ongoing monitoring of trauma patients

Indicator (Numerator): Trauma patients with blood pressure, pulse, respiration, and Glasgow Coma Scale (GCS) documented in the ED record on arrival and hourly until inpatient admission to operating room or intensive care unit, death, or transfer to another care facility (hourly GCS needed only if altered state of consciousness)

TR-3 *Indicator Focus:* Airway management of comatose trauma patients
Indicator (Numerator): Comatose patients discharged from the ED prior to the establishment of a mechanical airway

TR-4 *Indicator Focus:* Timeliness of diagnostic testing
Indicator (Numerator): Trauma patients with diagnosis of intracranial injury and altered state of consciousness upon ED arrival receiving initial head computerized tomography scan greater than two hours after ED arrival

TR-5 *Indicator Focus:* Timeliness of surgical intervention for adult head injury
Indicator (Numerator): Trauma patients with diagnosis of extradural or subdural brain hemorrhage undergoing craniotomy greater than four hours after ED arrival (excluding intracranial pressure monitoring) subcategorized by pediatric or adult patients

TR-6 *Indicator Focus:* Timeliness of surgical intervention for orthopedic injuries
Indicator (Numerator): Trauma patients with open fractures of the long bones as a result of blunt trauma receiving initial surgical treatment greater than eight hours after ED arrival

TR-7 *Indicator Focus:* Timeliness of surgical intervention for abdominal injuries
Indicator (Numerator): Trauma patients with diagnosis of

laceration of the liver or spleen requiring surgery and undergoing laparotomy greater than two hours after ED arrival, subcategorized by pediatric or adult patients

TR-8 ***Indicator Focus:*** Surgical decision making for abdominal gunshot wounds and/or stab wounds
Indicator (Numerator): Trauma patients undergoing laparotomy for wounds penetrating the abdominal wall subcategorized by gunshot and/or stab wounds

TR-9 ***Indicator Focus:*** Timeliness of patient transfers
Indicator (Numerator): Trauma patients transferred from initial receiving hospital to another acute care facility within six hours from ED arrival to ED departure

TR-10 ***Indicator Focus:*** Surgical decision making for orthopedic injuries
Indicator (Numerator): Adult trauma patients with femoral diaphyseal fractures treated by a nonfixation technique

TR-11 ***Indicator Focus:*** Clinical decision making for potentially preventable deaths
Indicator (Numerator): Intrahospital mortality of trauma patients—with one or more of the following conditions—who did not undergo a procedure for the condition: tension pneumothorax, hemoperitoneum, hemothoraces, ruptured aorta, pericardial tamponade, and epidural or subdural hemorrhage

TR-12 ***Indicator Focus:*** Systems necessary for obtaining autopsies for trauma victims
Indicator (Numerator): Trauma patients who expired within 48 hours of ED arrival for whom an autopsy was performed

Medication Use Indicators

MU-1 *Indicator Focus:* Individualizing dosage
Indicator (Numerator): Inpatients older than 65 years in whom creatinine clearance has been estimated

MU-2 *Indicator Focus:* Individualizing dosage
Indicator (Numerator): Inpatients receiving parenteral aminoglycosides who have a measured aminoglycoside serum level

MU-3 *Indicator Focus:* Reviewing the order
Indicator (Numerator): New medication orders prompting consultation by the pharmacist with physician or nurse subcategorized by orders changed

MU-4 *Indicator Focus:* Timing of medication administration
Indicator (Numerator): Patients receiving intravenous prophylactic antibiotics within two hours before the first surgical incision

MU-5 *Indicator Focus:* Accuracy of medication dispensing and administration
Indicator (Numerator): Number of reported significant medication errors

MU-6 *Indicator Focus:* Informing the patient about the medication
Indicator (Numerator): Inpatients with principal and/or other diagnoses of insulin-dependent diabetes mellitus who demonstrate self-blood-glucose monitoring and self-administration of insulin before discharge or are referred for postdischarge follow-up for diabetes management

MU-7 *Indicator Focus:* Monitoring patient response
Indicator (Numerator): Inpatients receiving digoxin, theophylline, phenytoin, or lithium who have no corre-

sponding measured drug levels or whose highest measured level exceeds a specific limit

MU-8 ***Indicator Focus:*** Monitoring patient response
Indicator (Numerator): Inpatients receiving warfarin or intravenous therapeutic heparin who also receive Vitamin K, protamine sulfate, or fresh frozen plasma

MU-9 ***Indicator Focus:*** Reporting adverse drug reactions (ADRs)
Indicator (Numerator): ADRs reported through the hospital's ADR-reporting system analyzed by method of reporting (spontaneous or retrospective medical record abstraction), type of ADR (dose related or non-dose related), and time of occurrence (before admission or during hospitalization)

MU-10 ***Indicator Focus:*** Reviewing complete drug regimen
Indicator (Numerator): Inpatients receiving more than one type of oral benzodiazepine simultaneously

MU-11 ***Indicator Focus:*** Reviewing complete drug regimen
Indicator (Numerator): Inpatients with seven or more prescribed medications on discharge

MU-12 ***Indicator Focus:*** Overall performance of medication use system
Indicator (Numerator): Patients younger than 25 years with a principal discharge diagnosis of bronchoconstrictive pulmonary disease, who are readmitted to the hospital or visit the emergency department within 15 days of discharge due to an exacerbation of their principal diagnosis

Infection Control Indicators

IC-1 ***Indicator Focus:*** Surgical wound infection
Indicator (Numerator): Selected inpatient and outpatient surgical procedures complicated by a wound infection during hospitalization or postdischarge

IC-2 *Indicator Focus:* Postoperative pneumonia
Indicator (Numerator): Selected inpatient surgical procedures complicated by the onset of pneumonia during hospitalization but not beyond ten postoperative days

IC-3 *Indicator Focus:* Urinary catheter usage
Indicator (Numerator): Selected surgical procedures on inpatients who are catheterized during the perioperative period

IC-4 *Indicator Focus:* Ventilator pneumonia
Indicator (Numerator): Ventilated inpatients who develop pneumonia

IC-5 *Indicator Focus:* Postpartum endometritis
Indicator (Numerator): Inpatients who develop endometritis following cesarean section, followed until discharge

IC-6 *Indicator Focus:* Concurrent surveillance of primary bloodstream infection
Indicator (Numerator): Inpatients with a central or umbilical line who develop primary bloodstream infection

IC-7 *Indicator Focus:* Medical record abstraction of primary bloodstream infection
Indicator (Numerator): Inpatients with a central or umbilical line and primary bloodstream infection, analyzed by method of identification

IC-8 *Indicator Focus:* Employee health program
Indicator (Numerator): Hospital staff who have been immunized for measles (rubeola) or are known to be immune

Home Infusion Therapy Indicators

Home Infusion Therapy Patient Population: Individuals for whom a home care agency has orders to administer, assess, monitor, maintain, or evaluate for infusion therapy. For the purposes of this indicator set infusion therapy includes parenteral nutrition, enteral therapy, immunotherapy/biological response modifiers, antibiotic therapy, pain management, blood products, and chemotherapy.

IT-1   **Indicator Focus:** Unscheduled inpatient admission by type of therapy

       Indicator (Numerator): Patients/clients receiving home infusion therapy who have an unscheduled inpatient admission to an acute care facility, during the designated reporting period, subcategorized by reason for admission

IT-2   **Indicator Focus:** Discontinued infusion therapy by type of therapy

       Indicator (Numerator): Courses of infusion therapy discontinued before prescribed completion, during the designated reporting period, subcategorized by reason for discontinuation

IT-3   **Indicator Focus:** Interruption in infusion therapy by type of therapy

       Indicator (Numerator): Total number of interruptions in infusion therapy, during the designated reporting period, subcategorized by reason for interruption in therapy

IT-4   **Indicator Focus:** Prevention and surveillance of infection by type of therapy

       Indicator (Numerator): Total number of suspected or confirmed catheter-related infections in patients/clients with central lines, for which the catheter is removed or antibiotics (oral or parenteral) are ordered, during the designated reporting period, subcategorized by type of central line catheter, number of lumens, and type of infection

IT-5 ***Indicator Focus:*** Reporting adverse drug reactions (ADRs)
Indicator (Numerator): Total number of suspected or
confirmed ADRs experienced by infusion therapy patients/
clients, during the designated reporting period, subcategorized by the type and severity of ADR and by drug class

IT-6 ***Indicator Focus:*** Patient/client monitoring and appropriate intervention
Indicator (Numerator): Patients/clients receiving total
parenteral nutrition and/or enteral therapy who have an
identified goal weight and are achieving or maintaining
desired weight, during the designated reporting period

ADDITIONAL INDICATORS APPROVED
FOR HOSPITAL USE

The following indicators have undergone alpha and/or beta testing
in the Joint Commission indicator development and testing process
and are recommended for internal hospital use only. (These indicators will not be included in the indicator monitoring system because
of difficulties in collecting comparable data across organizations.)

Additional Anesthesia Indicators

AN-A Patients with a discharge diagnosis of fulminant pulmonary
edema developed during procedures involving anesthesia
administration or within one postprocedure day of a
procedure's conclusion

AN-B Patients diagnosed with an aspiration pneumonitis occurring
during procedures involving anesthesia administration or
within two postprocedure days of a procedure's conclusion

AN-C Patients developing a postural headache within four
postprocedure days following procedures involving spinal
or epidural anesthesia administration

AN-D Patients experiencing a dental injury during procedures
involving anesthesia care

AN-E   Patients experiencing an ocular injury during procedures involving anesthesia care

AN-F   Unplanned admission of patients to the hospital within two postprocedure days following outpatient procedures involving anesthesia

AN-G   Unplanned admission of patients to an intensive care unit within two postprocedure days of procedures involving anesthesia administration and with intensive care unit stay greater than one day

Additional Obstetric Indicators

OB-A   Intrahospital neonatal deaths of infants with a birthweight of 750–999 grams born in a hospital with an NICU

OB-B   Maternal readmissions within 14 days of delivery

OB-C   Intrahospital maternal deaths occurring within 42 days postpartum

OB-D   Infants with a birthweight less than 1,800 grams delivered in a hospital without an NICU

OB-E   Neonates transferred from a non-NICU hospital to an NICU hospital

OB-F   Patients with excessive maternal blood loss

Additional Cardiovascular Indicators

CV-A *Indicator Focus:* Specific complication of CABG as a means of assessing the management of CABG patients *Indicator (Numerator):* Patients undergoing isolated CABG procedures returning to the operating room for treatment of postoperative thoracic bleeding subcategorized by presence or absence of thrombolytic therapy received within 48 hours prior to CABG

CV-B **Indicator Focus:** Specific complication of CABG as a
means of assessing multiple aspects of CABG care
Indicator (Numerator): Intraoperative or postoperative
cerebrovascular accident in patients undergoing isolated
CABG procedure

CV-C ***Indicator Focus:*** Effectiveness of PTCA
Indicator (Numerator): Patients with repeat PTCA of the
same lesion occurring within 72 hours of the most recent
PTCA subcategorized by emergent and nonemergent status
of original PTCA

CV-D ***Indicator Focus:*** Specific complication of PTCA as a means
of assessing multiple aspects of PTCA care
Indicator (Numerator): Patients with post-PTCA complications at femoral or brachial artery insertion site subcategorized by thrombolytic therapy within 48 hours prior
to PTCA

CV-E ***Indicator Focus:*** Management of thrombolytic therapy in
patients with acute MI
Indicator (Numerator): Hemorrhagic complications in
patients receiving thrombolytic therapy for acute MI
subcategorized by complications occurring to patients prior
to discharge from the institution initiating therapy and
posttransfer complications occurring to patients receiving
therapy prior to transfer

Additional Oncology Indicators

ON-A ***Indicator Focus:*** Availability of specific data needed for
diagnosis
Indicator (Numerator): Presence of a written pathology
report in the medical record of the treating institution
documenting the pathologic diagnosis of patients receiving initial treatment for primary lung, colorectal, or
female breast cancer

ON-B *Indicator Focus:* Symptomatic and/or palliative care
Indicator (Numerator): Systematic initial assessment of pain for all patients hospitalized due to metastatic lung, colorectal, or female breast cancer with pain

ON-C *Indicator Focus:* Use of clinical staging
Indicator (Numerator): Presence of documented AJCC clinical staging in the medical record prior to the first course of therapy for female patients with primary breast cancer

ON-D *Indicator Focus:* Use of multimodal therapy in treatment and follow-up
Indicator (Numerator): Treatment of female patients with primary invasive AJCC clinical Stage I or II breast cancer by excisional biopsy, segmental mastectomy, or quadrantectomy without radiation therapy

ON-E **Indicator Focus:** Use of psychosocial support for patient follow-up
Indicator (Numerator): Referral to support or rehabilitation groups or provision of psychosocial support for female patients with primary breast cancer

ON-F *Indicator Focus:* Patient education
Indicator (Numerator): Patients undergoing resection for primary colorectal cancer with enterostomy present at discharge who demonstrate understanding of enterostomy care and management instructions

Additional Trauma Indicators

TR-A *Indicator Focus:* Communication between EMS and ED
Indicator (Numerator): Copy of ambulance run report(s) not present with ED medical record for trauma patients transported by prehospital EMS personnel

TR-B ***Indicator Focus:*** Trauma patient assessments in the emergency department
Indicator (Numerator): Trauma patients admitted through the ED with inpatient discharge diagnosis of cervical spine injury not indicated in admission diagnosis

TR-C ***Indicator Focus:*** Emergency department decision making
Indicator (Numerator): Death of trauma patients with discharge diagnosis of closed pelvic fracture who receive transfusions of greater than six units of blood

TR-D ***Indicator Focus:*** Clinical decision making for surgical intervention
Indicator (Numerator): Trauma patients receiving initial abdominal, thoracic, vascular, or cranial surgery (excluding orthopedic, plastic, and hand surgery) more than 24 hours after ED arrival

TR-E ***Indicator Focus:*** Use of blood products
Indicator (Numerator): Transfusion of platelets and/or fresh frozen plasma within 24 hours of ED arrival in adult trauma patients receiving less than eight units of packed red blood cells or whole blood

TR-F ***Indicator Focus:*** Effectiveness of surgical intervention
Indicator (Numerator): Return of trauma patients to the operating room within 48 hours of completion of initial surgery

TR-G ***Indicator Focus:*** Clinical decision making for femoral shaft fractures
Indicator (Numerator): Trauma patients with femoral diaphyseal fractures that are not associated with other injuries who do not receive physical therapy or rehabilitation therapy

Index